PSYCHOANALYSIS AND HIDDEN NARRATIVE IN FILM

Psychoanalysis and Hidden Narrative in Film proposes a way of constructing hidden psychological narratives of popular films and novels. Instead of offering interpretations of classic films, Trevor C. Pederson recognizes that the psychoanalytic tradition began with making sense of the seemingly inconsequential. Here he turns his attention to popular films like Joel Schumacher's *The Lost Boys* (1987). While masterworks like *Psycho* (1960) are not the object of interpretation, Hitchcock's film is used as a skeleton key. The revelation that Norman Bates' character had been his mother all along, suggests a framework of reading a film as having symptom characters who are excised to create a latent plot. The symptom character's behavior or inter-relations are then transcribed to an ego character. This is a shift in the tradition of literary doubling from hermeneutic intuition to a formal methodology that generates data for the unconscious.

Pederson continues the project of unifying competing schools into a single model of mind and offers clinical examples from his own practice for all its terms. Psychodynamic techniques that emphasize the importance of working with the body, the id, and the ubiquity of repetition are introduced. A return to Freud's structural theory, in which complexes are anchored in the stages of superego development, is used to carefully plot and explain the social nature of the superego and its relation to authority in society (secondary narcissism) and the otherworldly (primary narcissism). Discrete phases of superego development and their ties to both the social and the id revive the grand promises of classical psychoanalysis to link with every field in the humanities.

Psychoanalysis and Hidden Narrative in Film will appeal to psychoanalysts and psychoanalytic psychotherapists as well as scholars of film studies and literature interested in using a psychoanalytic approach and ideas in their work.

Trevor C. Pederson is a licensed professional counsellor and psychoanalyst in private practice in Laramie, Wyoming. His 2015 book *The Economics of Libido: Psychic Bisexuality, the Superego, and the Centrality of the Oedipus Complex* won the 2016 Gradiva Award for Best Book.

PSYCHOANALYSIS AND HIDDEN NARRATIVE IN FILM

Reading the Symptom

Trevor C. Pederson

Routledge
Taylor & Francis Group
LONDON AND NEW YORK

First published 2019
by Routledge
2 Park Square, Milton Park, Abingdon, Oxon OX14 4RN

and by Routledge
711 Third Avenue, New York, NY 10017

Routledge is an imprint of the Taylor & Francis Group, an informa business

British Library Cataloguing in Publication Data
A catalogue record for this book is available from the British Library

Library of Congress Cataloging in Publication Data
A catalog record for this book has been requested

ISBN: 978-1-138-30709-4 (hbk)
ISBN: 978-1-138-30714-8 (pbk)
ISBN: 978-1-315-14223-4 (ebk)

Typeset in Bembo
by Swales & Willis Ltd, Exeter, Devon, UK

To Arielle and Jonah. For all the mornings.

CONTENTS

ACKNOWLEDGMENTS

I would like to thank Julia Ivanova for sharing her love of film with me. I would like to thank Mike Eigen for his continued encouragement to find my voice. I also have an appreciation for Jon Mills and Arnie Richards for their openness and ideas. Also, thanks to Julia Whyde for her comments, and Siamak Movahedi for his patience with me.

My gratitude to Kate Hawes and Charles Bath at Routledge.

I would like to thank all the patients with whom I have worked and who let me act as their psychopomp and confessor. To see you find your courage and share your pain with me has opened my eyes to more than I had dreamt of finding.

In the clinical vignettes, I have left out names and changed details to protect anonymity. Only they will be able to recognize who they are.

INTRODUCTION

In film there is a living unconscious. The subtleties of a disordered personality can be captured, and the conflicts between characters can be enhanced by cinematography to create a felt sense for how powerful or seductive the pain in our relationships can be. Despite the value of articulating this, the aim of this book is to show how a return to Freudian psychoanalysis is capable of giving us much, much more. As one critic of psychoanalytic criticism puts it:

> Psychoanalytic readings purport to show the meaning behind the text that is concealed by its manifest content, but it is not clear that this is what psychoanalytic readings of Hollywood cinema achieve . . . [A]rguably, far from providing an objective code to unlock the real (hidden) meaning of the text, psychoanalytic criticism quite frequently describes what is going on at the surface of it . . . However, if this is the case, the psychoanalytic critic posing as theorist erroneously claims for himself the insight that rightly belongs to the text itself.
>
> *(Allen, 1999, p. 142)*

Allen is skeptical about how much insight psychoanalytic critics bring to a text, as opposed to using the insight on the surface of the text to illustrate one of their theories. Others are not as kind. If literary critics do not dispute the status of psychoanalysis as a coherent model of understanding, many dismiss the applications of it as boring. One sees a character attach a lot of importance to a non-human object and calls it a transitional object; one sees a woman seductively portrayed and calls it the masculine gaze; one finds a triangle with two men and a woman and labels it oedipal. Others search for images or references to penises or feces, and still others do wordplay with the names and places of the text—lending to the impression that psychoanalysis is a silly game for the vulgar or overly erudite.

I would side with Allen in suggesting that the mere description of surface phenomena in the text is simply a game of matching, and that this game leaves the text's valuable latent content unearthed. However, while Allen takes aim at predominately Lacanian based criticism (Metz, 1982; Mulvey, 1989; Doane, 1991; Žižek, 1992), he does not acknowledge a parallel tradition that does build latent content of psychological significance: the psychoanalytic criticism of the double. Plots of the double, trafficking as they do in repressed psychological content actively represented through double figurations, bypasses what has long been perceived as a failing of the Lacanian analysis of film. We are given latent insight into how a character feels, and this can sometimes be used to explain idiosyncratic behaviors or moments when the character is acting "out of character."

I will argue that there are three schools of double scholarship. It begins with the fantastic, or supernatural double who is either a physical duplicate (doppelgänger) of the protagonist's body, looking identical to the protagonist, or manifests in one body being controlled by multiple personalities (ex. Dr. Jekyll and Mr. Hyde). Early psychoanalytic critics like Otto Rank (1941, 1971) also point to familial ties, or "blood," as providing a shared essence that can make family members into doubles who represent pathological feelings or socially unacceptable desires. The first school of double scholarship is therefore built upon a supernatural relation to the body or shared essence through family.

The next wave of scholarship goes beyond the body. From the foundation of the moral opposition between characters, and with a subtler textual analysis, the criticism frees itself from the ties to the protagonist's body or family. Doubles can now be found in potentially any other character in the text. Interestingly, one of the first examples of doubles of this kind comes from Freud (1916) who builds the case that Lady Macbeth expresses the bad conscience of Macbeth. He writes:

> [W]ith Macbeth and Lady Macbeth . . . it would of course be pointless to regard her as an independent character and seek to discover the motives for her change . . . the germs of fear which break out in Macbeth on the night of the murder do not develop further in *him* but in *her*. It is he who has the hallucination of the dagger before the crime; but it is she who afterwards falls ill of a mental disorder. It is he who after the murder hears the cry in the house: "Sleep no more! Macbeth does murder sleep . . ." and so "Macbeth shall sleep no more"; but we never hear that *he* slept no more, while the Queen, as we see, rises from her bed and, talking in her sleep, betrays her guilt. It is he who stands helpless with bloody hands, lamenting that "all great Neptune's ocean" will not wash them clean, while she comforts him: "A little water clears us of this deed"; but later it is she who washes her hands for a quarter of an hour and cannot get rid of the bloodstains: "All the perfumes of Arabia will not sweeten this little hand." Thus what he feared in his pangs of conscience is fulfilled in her; she becomes all remorse and he all defiance. Together they exhaust the possibilities of reaction to the crime, like two disunited parts of a single psychical individuality, and it may be that they are both copied from a single prototype.
>
> *(ibid., pp. 323–324)*

The manifest plot of the play lacks a sufficient motivation for Lady Macbeth's forceful pathological reactions, but textual clues suggest the interpretation that these reactions are a better fit for Macbeth himself. This kind of close reading illustrates how the next school of double scholarship emerges. The two central critics of this period are Rogers (1970) and Keppler (1972). The former carries on the psychoanalytic tradition and follows Rank in pointing to the concept of narcissism as the explanatory factor in the *decomposition* that allows one character to express another's antisocial impulses. The other major critic, Keppler, provides additional insight here and, instead of psychoanalytic concepts, he holds that this kind of double "represents a certain stage of development . . . *within* the first self's own lifetime" (Keppler, 1972, p. 172). In contrast to Rogers, Keppler also pays closer attention to textual differences, such as whether the double is given objective status by being registered as a fully separate character in the narrative or as a subjective self that may just reference the psychology of the protagonist (i.e. be a projection). Keppler is skeptical of psychoanalysis and hopes that a careful study of doubles will add to psychological knowledge instead of being explained away by it. Despite the divergences, both men recognize that some of the authors are not conscious of the creation of the latent doubles in their stories and that a psychological interpretation of their creation is needed.

The third school of the criticism of the double is based upon feminist literature that sees the double emerge from the oppressive patriarchal social order. Gilbert and Gubar's seminal *The Madwoman in the Attic* (1979) is a prime example of this school. Instead of individual repression, gender roles and the limits they place upon characters are posited as the cause of the double. "[T]he striking coherence we noticed in literature by women could be explained," they write, "by a common, female impulse to struggle free from social and literary confinement through strategic redefinitions of self, art, and society" (ibid., pp. xi–i). The antisocial impulses of Bertha, the secret wife of Rochester in Bronte's *Jane Eyre* (1847), for example, can be the emotional expression of the titular character when she encounters her own frustrations with Rochester. Her internalization of a feminine role would make such aggression unseemly, necessitating the appearance of Bertha as a double. Readings from this wave of scholarship are indifferent to the psychological understanding of the double and, instead, seem best understood as viewing the protagonist as a double of the patriarchal social order, which unduly limits them.

The double scholarship of the second and third school works with the text to say something about a character beyond a surface description of the text's action. We are given an insight into aspects of the protagonist's emotional life through the externalization of part of his or her personality. This makes double scholarship potentially the start of an answer to critics of psychoanalytic interpretations. The issue is that hitherto, double criticism does not decode the "real (hidden) meaning of the text" (Allen, 1999, p. 42), but only offers insights into one or more characters. The methodology that I will advance is to build a whole latent plot and provide hidden narrative that will explain idiosyncratic aspects of the manifest plot. I will return to this in a moment.

In assessing the literary tradition of scholarship on the double, my primary interest is in critics who relate their findings to a psychoanalytic framework. I will use their criticism to develop the important trans-historical insights into personality found in the psychoanalytic model of mind. This will either come from the explication of how the doppelgänger relates to concepts like narcissism and the uncanny, or by disagreement with the representation of psychoanalysis that a critic gives. However, I acknowledge, especially with the manifest double, that there has to be a dialectic between the psychological inputs and the cultural ones.

Broadly, any cultural movement, whether philosophical, religious, or artistic, will define itself against what has come before, or potentially cross-pollinate. In *The Divided Self: A Perspective on the Literature of the Victorians* (1969), Masao Miyoshi argues that the Romantics, in defining themselves against the Gothic tradition, continue the questioning of self-identity begun with the literary tradition of the Gothic. The Gothic villain shows self-consciousness of his antisocial impulses, the darkness within him, which leads to a new formulation of this darkness of identity through the division of the double. In *The Doppelgänger: Double Visions in German Literature* (1996), Andrew Webber investigates the "crisis" engendered by movements like German idealist philosophy and mesmerism though the writings and letters of the period's authors. The uniqueness of the period's philosophy held to be the foundation of the double, and Webber argues that the double should be viewed a as post-Romantic figure. It is Romantic, but with irony (ibid., p 11). Lastly, John Herdman in *The Double in Nineteenth-Century Fiction* (1990) holds that the double is a central romantic image, but sees cross-pollination from religion. For Herdman, the "Christian belief in the final resurrection of the body, a body different in substance from the physical body . . . could not fail to be richly suggestive" (ibid., p. 3). Whether directly from Christian belief, ideas of the occult, or notions at work in the mesmerism of the time, he sees the double as having to register the theological question of the dualism in the nature of humans: the spirit and the flesh. I will not be reviewing the work of these critics, but I want to acknowledge the input they see from the sociological register.

After this review, I will proceed to build upon the established methodologies of double interpretation. Again, the key advancement is the creation of a whole latent plot as opposed to just finding to whom the inconsistent emotion or psychological content is displaced. In my readings, I refer to the double as the "symptom character," because in its manifestation of the primary, or ego character's latent desires, the symptom character resembles what Freud (1900) divined in his concept of a symptom (pp. 569–570). A symptom both allows the expression of an unconscious desire and, at the same time, only reveals this desire in hidden form. This insight is visible on the surface of several texts. For example, both Alfred Hitchcock's *Psycho* (1960) and David Fincher's *Fight Club* (1999) end with the revelation that one of the characters did not exist and that the protagonist/antagonist was responsible for the actions of their double. In *Psycho*, Norman Bates' mother had been Norman all along, and he was responsible for the murder central to the plot of the film. These endings encourage a re-watching of the film, with an eye to how the ego character managed to perform all of the actions attributed to the symptom character in addition to his own. In my readings of films that do not make these endings explicit, I perform the same interpretative work as such re-watchings. I do not suggest, by this mode of interpretation, that such endings are missing nor do I imply that the films are inherently flawed. Instead, I mean to suggest that the psychological content that is made explicit by the endings of films like *Psycho* or *Fight Club* is nonetheless also present in films that make the formal decision to keep their latent doubles hidden.

The film that I will analyze in this book, *The Lost Boys* (1987), was chosen because it is the film from which this methodology was born. The irony that I will not be offering an interpretation of a major film like *Psycho*, but instead will argue that it manifestly offers the interpretative key to a minor film like *The Lost Boys*, is not lost on me. However, one of the charms that psychoanalysis accustoms one to is that content that is often seen as beneath the dignity of serious investigation, such as dreams, slips of the tongue, etc., often has relevance for the open-minded. I will be presenting the analysis of *The Lost Boys* with an eye for the logic of how the five-step procedure of the symptom reading suggested itself to me. This cult classic was a popular film that, as in the Romantic and Gothic traditions before it, contains supernatural elements. These supernatural elements, along with the split plot structure between the movie's two brothers, provided the initial support for building a latent plot. However, as I will illustrate in the conclusion of this book and subsequent volumes, neither the supernatural elements in the plot nor the split plot structure are needed to perform the symptom reading.

Along with formalizing the new methodology, I will be offering a partial explication of Freud's model of mind. In *The Economics of the Libido: Psychic Bisexuality, the Superego, and the Centrality of the Oedipus Complex* (2015), I argue that Freud gives us an axis of vertical development in the superego and a horizontal axis in psychic bisexuality. The latter, psychic bisexuality, is based upon the notion that there are "two sets of emotional impulses . . . opposed to each other . . . impulses of an affectionate and submissive nature, but also hostile and defiant ones" (Freud, 1923a, p. 85). Freud holds that under the cultural ideals of gender, personality has both an active and passive pole that relate to biological sex. However, he also holds that every human being has motivational and character patterns of the opposite sex or defenses against them. He writes:

> In human beings pure masculinity or femininity is not to be found either in a psychological or a biological sense. Every individual on the contrary displays a mixture of the character-traits belonging to his own and to the opposite sex; and he shows a combination of activity and passivity whether or not these last character-traits tally with his biological ones.
>
> *(Freud, 1905, p. 219 fn; see also Freud, 1933, p. 105)*

Freud aligns the female sex with passivity and masochism in some places, and cautions against doing so in other places. Psychic bisexuality was never fully elaborated in his work, but one finds the seeds for many interesting ideas there. I will wait until the next book to fully introduce these ideas, since there is already enough theoretical ground to cover. For this book, I will make general references to the two poles of personality: an active pole that registers competition, the desirability of power, and dynamics of superiority/inferiority, and a passive pole that registers the desire to restore harmony or oneness with others, the desirability of belonging, and dynamics of inclusion/exclusion. Although my focus will one-sidedly be on power dynamics in Chapter 5, I want my reader to know that this is far from being the full story.

The main focus of the psychoanalytic theory in Chapter 5 will be on the vertical axis of superego development. I will go beyond what I introduced in *The Economics of Libido* (2015) to provide clinical examples for the stages and split them up into different phases. Generally, Freud (1921) draws our attention to the binary of people with a high ego ideal and people with a low ego ideal. In the latter, "the ego has often preserved its earlier narcissistic self-complacency . . . [and] the individuals concerned . . . give an impression of greater force and of more freedom of libido" (pp. 129–130). In other words, such an individual shows more confidence, without necessarily having all the skills, knowledge, or expertise that others do. Additionally, this can translate into the individual feeling entitled to be a boss, leader, or authority figure even when others are more competent, or into making a virtue of risk-taking and following one's gut, without having all the available facts or training. Others are often impressed by such an individual's confidence. Often the rhetorical approach of the individual with a low ego ideal will resonate more than someone who tries to reference competence in the field by getting into the details. In contrast, an active individual with a high ego ideal has a more developed sense of shame. This sense of shame is related to conscientiousness, a sense of wanting to be seen as competent in one's field of work, or anxiety that one's work will be judged as inferior or found wanting.

This high and low ego ideal and its relation to authority is central to the Oedipus complex in psychoanalytic theory. Contrary to popular understanding, the Oedipus complex's clinical relevance rarely involves a sexual interest in the opposite-sexed parent. This strange and very pathological relation, such as the one depicted between the fictional Norman Bates and his mother, are the exception, and not the rule. Instead, the Oedipus complex is more often expressed through relations with the *parental-substitute* and not the actual parent. Freud (1924) is explicit that in "the Oedipus complex . . . [the parent's] personal significance for the superego recedes into the background" and "the imagos they leave behind . . . link [to] the influences of teachers and authorities" (pp. 167–168). Between different levels of authority in society, the mediating factor is care for one's reputation or the reputation of the family (or company, work group, etc.). A common conversation I have with many criminal patients concerns a period of time during their teenage years in which they stopped caring about getting good grades or embarrassing their families by getting in trouble. The importance of reputation, shame at its loss, and the need to have a reputation of importance is what is at stake. In other words, through interaction with caregivers during psychosexual development, the child comes to form inputs that later correspond to different levels of authority in society.[1]

The ego ideal is a non-moral aspect of the superego, which is formed from the parental imagos that are internalized for each stage of psychosexual development. For the ego ideal, there is a sense of increasing authority regarding the wealthy, the upper classes, the experts of different professions, the presidents and leaders of a society, and the world-historical individuals. The ego ideal references these levels of authority and the corresponding sense of inferiority, self-hate, or self-criticism of increasing magnitudes that one feels for not attaining the success that these authorities possess. The conscience, or moral aspect of the superego, references shame at ethical transgressions that vary in magnitude and run parallel with this increasing authority.[2] Breaking folkways is not as egregious as breaking mores and laws, and crimes can reach the level at which they become heinous, monstrous, and evil. As with the self-criticism of the ego ideal, the conscience can respond to such ethical transgressions with an increasing tension of remorse, shamefulness, or self-hate. These two aspects together illustrate how an individual can take himself as object, or observe himself in a way that is rife with tension and conflict, as well as how he is primarily related to the social body. The superego is how Freud includes the Other in his model of mind.

In Chapter 5 I will provide a full explication of Freud's four-stage model of authority and object relations, and the different phases of each stage. I will seek to build consensus between analysts from different schools of psychoanalysis and use many clinical examples to operationalize the theory. However, as mentioned above, these levels of Being will only be examined narrowly and in relation to the active pole of the personality with a focus on traits like ambition, competitiveness, and power. Clinical examples that reference the passive pole will also be examined, but its formal introduction will be in the subsequent volume.

It is important to mention a few things about the clinical examples that I will be giving in this book. Before I begin the literature review, the first chapter will show the innovations in clinical technique that I have made due to the requirements of short-term therapy. They are psychodynamic techniques that build on eye movement desensitization and reprocessing (EMDR) and sensorimotor approaches. Instead of interpretation, the techniques have the patient associate to material he or she produces; the patient therefore gives the clinician the relevant material from his or her past. In some cases, the patient and analyst co-create a fantasy that allows for the relevant level of Being, authority, or power of the parental imago to be illustrated in what can appear as a much more mundane relationship. In turn, the parental or sibling imagos placed on others through the superego are tied to specific anxiety states, idiosyncratic forms of aggression and affection, and particular bodily zones and symbols. This content is related to what is known as the id in psychoanalytic theory, and I will show how pervasive the id is in the technique. Ultimately, I hope to give my reader the sense that doubling in literary criticism is not just a textual phenomenon, but also a common feature of clinical work. Many people are essentially projecting an injured part of themselves onto another person, repeating with someone new the hurt that they received from a parent, sibling, or their substitutes.

Because of our shared trans-historical, psychosexual development, these ego injuries and traumas resonate with the relevant imago in other people. People are often unconsciously attracted to each other in order to repeat their hurt or injury, or in order to give another the same pain that they had experienced. As Freud (1917a) writes,

> our mind is not a simple thing; on the contrary, it is a hierarchy of superordinated and subordinated agencies, a labyrinth of impulses striving independently of one another towards action, corresponding with the multiplicity of instincts and of relations with the external world, many of which are antagonistic to one another and incompatible.
>
> *(p. 141)*

Freud (1917a) compares this view of the mind, of seeing the ego or "the I" in parts, to the revolutions of thought found in Copernicus and Darwin. As I progress through the chapters, I will begin with more general remarks about this orientation and the structural agencies involved. By the fifth chapter I will move into the analysis of the Oedipus complex and the oedipal castration complex that stretches across the four stages of psychosexual development in Freud's work. The vertical axis of development is an important feature of the later analysis of the symptom reading. It is necessary to illustrate the clinical phenomenon of regression, or introversion of libido, which will show what is at stake for the protagonist of the *The Lost Boys*, Sam, once all the supernatural elements are excised in order to build the latent plot. Lastly, the conclusion will focus on the formalized five-step methodology, which will be tested and revised in the books to follow this one.[3]

I

Let me make a few disclaimers about the methodology that I will introduce. First, the latent meaning the symptom reading produces is in no way exhaustive, nor does it claim exclusivity. Just as there are several ways to interpret or utilize dreams, a narrative can be interpreted in several ways. Second, I have chosen to analyze films, but that does not mean the method only works with cinema. It can also be applied to literature or any medium that possesses a narrative. Third, the symptom reading can be performed by the layperson who is not well versed in psychoanalytic theory—though, I am sure that knowledge of theory might help to loosen the mind in order to make some connections. However, in many cases, knowing psychoanalysis "too well" can equally be a hindrance.

Lastly, after viewing *The Lost Boys*, I formulated a hypothesis that the "objective code" of the symptom reading is based upon the metapsychology of an individual's libidinal economy. People like narratives with which they can identify. For example, not everyone likes action movies, and those who do can identify with the motivations of the action heroes or villains because they share those same motivations (i.e. to compete with others, to achieve success, admiration, or recognition from others, to want to be the strongest and/or smartest, or most "potent," or feeling wronged or betrayed, wanting revenge, disregarding moral feelings because one is "an exception," etc.). Of course, there are certain mechanisms that interfere with this identification. For example, one can have an ego identification with, or an adverse reaction to, a parental-substitute or gender role. Similarly, certain sociological factors can shift identification and reaction. For example, a certain genre coming into fashion can increase spectatorship, and many can want to imitate it. But, all else being equal, one's motivational structure, or economics of libido, should have a major impact here. Upon performing the literature review, I was happy to see that Robert Rogers (1970) had already formulated this hypothesis and that my intuition was shared.

Individual viewers potentially identify with characters in a text, but the process of identification extends outward to the writer. The writer of the script also identifies with the central character(s), and when the writer's complexes, which are tied to anxiety or the need for punishment, come up in relation to the motivations given to the character, the writer externalizes them onto a double or symptom character. In this way, the enjoyment of the ego character is not reduced by the anxiety, the need for punishment, or tensions between what a person thinks they should be and what they are (i.e. the superego). Similarly, this should also work for the people who want to make the movie. They also identify with the narrative and, through the images and changes in dialogue, can contribute to the complex found in the film (and potentially decrease its expression). In the next book, I will begin to evaluate whether identification with the ego character and externalizing the behavior that leads to anxiety or displeasure can be taken as the cause of forming the symptom character, as appears to be the case with *The Lost Boys*.

II

I am skeptical that spending a lot of time on these introductory remarks and showing the clinical vignettes in the first chapter will do much to persuade a non-psychoanalyst of the validity of psychoanalysis. I would again like to direct them to *The Economics of Libido* (2015) for the explication of Wittgenstein's private language argument and the philosophical foundations that directed me to study psychoanalysis. My main interest, along with building on the model of mind in *The Economics of Libido* (2015), is to attract the reader who may have been repelled by psychoanalytic criticism in the past.

Psychologists or psychoanalysts do not have a monopoly on wisdom. A good critic using common language often gives a more satisfying reading than someone using theory. Good literary criticism, which is not historical research into the time period or potential influences on the writer, is possible when the critic discusses individual motivations and what appears troubling or illogical in the plot. The critic has a sense for actions or behaviors that are inconsistent with the type of person that a character has been portrayed as: those that appear "out of character." A good critic can criticize a narrative that did not develop a relationship enough to give the reader a sense of the magnitude of its importance or how it justifies certain character actions. This emotional intelligence (EQ) stands in contrast to the IQ of the pragmatist who can criticize the plot holes and failures of "common sense" in a zombie or action movie.

The common language approach will always remain the most important approach to appreciate the beauty and health of the text, and to point out its lack. The health found in the text resonates with the health of the critic, and, through variations of its theme, she can help others to a greater appreciation the text. Of course, text appreciation is also heightened by acknowledging the conventions it follows and breaks and its historical context; these elements add butter to the bread of what a fan hungers for in terms of appreciating a text.

However, I am not sharing the symptom reading as a method for the appreciation of the health and beauty of a text. The symptom reading deals in pathology and, as such, represents what Nietzsche would criticize as decadence. To this end, I will sometimes choose very bad films to interpret in future publications. The introduction of the symptom reading is primarily for the benefit of psychoanalysts. Doubling generates data for what can be repressed or dissociated, and once I introduce psychic bisexuality in the next book, the symptom reading will help with training the EQ or phenomenology of clinicians. By examining the different motivational structures of the horizontal axis, different nuclear complexes will be illustrated that will take us beyond naming every triangular interaction oedipal.

Still, I imagine that the most fanatical lovers of narrative—the schizoid types who can only love by turning something inside out and eventually killing it—may find some appeal in the symptom reading. To such literary critics, I hope this book can be a call beyond cleverness and move readers to once again experience some awe before the mystery of human psychology. But, maybe awe is not the right word—maybe I am just presenting glimpses of the human personality broken down into pieces and creating an annoying chaos with many unresolved aspects and angles. For those driven to have cleanliness, this approach may attract them; they will use their brooms to chase the rats out of the kitchen. There are many different types of people to be found in any culture. Bringing their motivations, attitudes, and style of relating into prominence, and to show the depth structures that underpin them, is what the symptom reading aims to do.

Notes

1 As we will come to see later, this also means authority beyond society that references reality principles that are found in Time and Space.
2 Shame and its relation to what Freud (1914a, p. 102; 1926a, p. 139) calls social anxiety, as a form of castration anxiety, has to be differentiated from the later form of full conscience that manifests guilt. This will be taken up in detail in Chapter 6.
3 The psychoanalytic model of mind is also up for revision and stands to be informed by the symptom reading as well.

1

NOTES ON THE PSYCHOANALYTIC ORIENTATION AND INNOVATIONS IN CLINICAL TECHNIQUE

> Of the three factors which we have recognized as being decisive for the success or otherwise of analytic treatment—the influence of traumas, the constitutional strength of the instincts and alterations of the ego . . . We can only say: "So muss denn doch die Hexe dran!" ["We must call the Witch to our help after all!" Goethe, *Faust*, Part I, Scene 6.]—the Witch Meta-psychology. Without meta-psychological speculation and theorizing—I had almost said "phantasying"—we shall not get another step forward. Unfortunately, here as elsewhere, what our Witch reveals is neither very clear nor very detailed.
>
> *(Freud, 1937, pp. 224–225)*

I would like to begin with some guiding remarks about where I see psychoanalysis today and how it has gotten here. From here I will discuss the general orientation of Freud's model of mind and then follow one thread of it, the idea of the characterologically based ambition. I will show how characterological ambition has been discussed by some psychoanalytic writers in order to illustrate the importance of the concept of the superego in Freud's work. Once I impart the grand sense of it that is found in Freud's writing, I will turn to introducing the clinical techniques that will be showcased in the vignettes throughout the book. Along with explaining how I came up with them, and how they are extensions of psychoanalytic theory, this chapter is meant to show how doubling is omnipresent in the clinic. When psychotherapists speak of personality disorders or characterological issues, very often it concerns the patient usurping the place of a parental imago that was formed in psychosexual development and projecting out the self—in effect identifying with another person who is now the person's double (i.e. projective identification). The individual now becomes his or her own ideal, or more precisely, the failure of this ideal and gives others the same pain that he or she received. Another important aspect of the technique is the use of the body, images, and symbols. Freud (1923b) famously writes that "[t]he ego is first and foremost a bodily ego; it is not merely a surface entity, but is itself the projection of a surface" (p. 26). However, before the body ego becomes the entire surface of the body, it relates to specific erotogenic zones or parts of the body, as well as to the breast of the mother. The recognition of this has allowed me to bypass some of the primitive defenses that block access to the repressed feelings of the initial ego injury with idealized others. Working with the introjection of symbols and images into bodily zones will show up in many of my vignettes.

Many who call themselves psychoanalysts have abandoned the Oedipus complex, metapsychology, and the model of mind that give psychoanalysis a foundation and a unique place among other therapeutic approaches. It is not difficult to see the roots of this in a dialectical relation with other discourses in the mid-twentieth century: psychopharmacology; postmodernism, and the valorization of freedom and evil. I do not believe it is a coincidence that they came into prominence after the social trauma of two World Wars. These discourses, in some ways, highlight areas that the classical model of mind either neglected or undertheorized. However, for some psychoanalysts, they have become an end in themselves—an epistemological block that prevents the reconciliation with classical theory. Some have given up research into subjectivity and the mind for research into the brain. Some have thrown out individual psychology, denied pre-discursive desire, or claimed that the psychoanalytic unconscious is co-created in the office with the analyst (as if it did not exist without the analyst there). Some have returned the rational ego to the position of "master of the house" and their references to freedom in the clinical encounter replace early findings of intrapsychic defenses. Leveraging the transference to force identifications with the "good habits" or structured life of the analyst becomes the aim instead of the liberation of the patient's own subjectivity.

Psychoanalysis began its fall from grace in the mid-twentieth century and the discourses that began to replace it, or were integrated with it, were far less challenging to the political status quo. There are economic elites who have the motivation to justify certain societal arrangements and inequalities. Such people pay psychologists and advertisers to help them "focus group" something in order to find the right meme for their propaganda campaigns. However, I do not think that this elite is as intelligent and farsighted as some believe, nor that they derive their power from secret societies of the past. Although I recognize their influence in class conflict, I would hold that their power is analogous to the rational ego who serves and rationalizes for its two masters: *the drives* in the id and ego, and *the identifications* in the ego and superego. In this light, it is more important to examine the social traumas of the World Wars, than the economic elite, if one wants to examine how psychoanalysis fell out of favor.

There were surely many soldiers who returned from the World Wars with PTSD. Both they and their families had the resulting need to valorize the importance of the war and give meaning to its chaos and death. A powerful discourse of free will and choosing to be on the side of good against evil is one such meaning. Additionally, the primitive defenses of PTSD that make one "shell-shocked," detached from feeling, hypervigilant, etc., put powerful impediments on the openness to new experiences, and the pursuit of happiness through love of friends, romantic partners, and one's profession. Instead, power and control dynamics are emphasized with an authoritarian codification of what is orthodoxy and what is heresy. Giving life meaning through choosing values, instead of "following one's instincts" was preached by many and passed on to their children. However, we know that this "autonomous choosing" is not openness and what really happens is that one forms ego identifications with authority figures and the worldviews from the groups to which they belong. Logic is evidenced in the rationalizations of why one's identifications are correct, and not in the open search for truth, nor the synthesis of ideas between several group identifications.

Freud's scientific naturalism, with its positions against religion and free will, came into strong conflict with the valorization of freedom and rational autonomy. The vast complexity of his model with its many subordinate and superordinate agencies that over-determine psychic acts and somatic behaviors became split. On one hand, it required too much openness and empathy, and outside the public discourse, determinism in the university became autistic. It eschewed phenomenology and subjectivity in favor of simple behavioristic conditioning and then for the power of genetics and "brain chemistry." On the other hand, the complex subjectivity in the psychoanalytic model also became histrionic in the university. It was externalized to the cultural level in the relativism and semiotics of postmodernism, and gender and group identities were valorized to the neglect of individual psychology. Within popular culture, Freudian ideas were slowly pushed back until psychology and the self-help industry began to teach people how to master their own house again through positive thinking. There is still the occasional glimmer of Freud, and a patient will come in and tell me that she thinks she has "daddy issues," for example, but many more patients bring up God, ideas of focusing on the positive and finding their gratitude, or some other mystical framework.

Psychoanalysis, for the practitioners who also identity with one of these other groups, is a therapeutic technique that is based upon transference, but the foundation of transference hangs in the air. The link to infantile sexuality, aggression, general childhood development, and an individual's functioning in the community, society, or the world at large is severed through this disconnect. Without the witch metapsychology, these analysts are mostly left to re-invent the wheel—coining new terms for concepts that already existed in the classical model of mind. Outside of such dubious projects, the other approach is to create a straw man of Freud, and other early analysts, in order to make an apology project for how psychoanalysis did not recognize the importance of the currently fashionable trends of thought in academia.

I do not wish to write a book that destroys, and would much rather build; as such, I will not dwell on these criticisms of the field. Anyway, other analysts like Mills (2012), have already done an impressive job at pointing out the lack of a foundation in contemporary psychoanalytic movements. While analysts like Richards (2015) have shown the authoritarian practices in psychoanalytic institutes that have led to dogmatism and the ideological transmission of knowledge.

Towards my end, I will be including several clinical vignettes to illustrate the empirical nature of psychoanalytic concepts. Most of these examples are not based upon transference to the analyst, but are based instead on the ubiquity of transference in human life. To understand this requires the concept of repetition through ego and object drives and the concept of the superego. For my purposes in this chapter, I will just give brief definitions and a few quotations to help orient my reader, but much more on these concepts will come later.

I

Transference is the replaying of relationships with parents, siblings, and important figures from one's past with the therapist. The hope is that the psychoanalyst does not actually replay the relationship with the patient, but instead interprets that the patient is trying to transfer the old relationship onto the analyst.[1] However, Freud (1925) is explicit that:

> [i]t must not be supposed, however, that transference is created by analysis and does not occur apart from it. Transference is merely uncovered and isolated by analysis. It is a universal phenomenon of the human mind, it decides the success of all medical influence, and in fact *dominates the whole of each person's relations to his human environment.*
>
> *(p. 42, emphasis added)*

Although Freud sees transference as omnipresent, it does not issue forth indiscriminately, nor does every relation to others involve ambivalence. The concept of the superego, in its aspect of the ego ideal, provides the structure for transference. In his study on group psychology, Freud (1921) expresses that the ego ideal links the individual to authority in the human environment, and the leaders that wield it, at various levels through a "double kind of tie . . . putting the object in the place of the ego ideal" (ibid., p. 130). This is thrown into sharper relief when one leaves the isolation of the analyst's office. In the office, patients can attribute many different estimates of power or authority to the analyst, but transference can become fickle once one steps outside of it. A group psychotherapist, can observe how the authority originally granted to her by members can be challenged and taken away if she does not properly handle defiance from a rival in the group. Additionally, the ebb and flow of political topics in group therapy will often put the facilitator in the place of having to answer for the errors or evils of greater authorities in society, as if she is a spokesperson for the government. Although one's authority can be diminished, or one can be perceived to have more of it than is realistic, transference is not randomly formed in society. It references a fairly stable classification of society being comprised of different classes.

Freud's argument for the centrality of transference, the superego, and the imagos from which they arise, is based upon his *Copernican Revolution* (Freud, 1917a). He holds that if we study the broken mind or the mind that has become rigid in pathology, we can get a glimpse into how the normal mind must work (Freud, 1933, pp. 58–59). When a paranoiac, for example, thinks that the end of the world is coming, that random people in public might want to fight him, that he is being hunted by the CIA, or that people are conspiring to ruin his reputation, different estimates of power/authority are in evidence here. Instead of saying that the mind is rational and mental illness belongs to chemical imbalance in the brain, or is a problem of the passions—associated with the body and trying to cloud the rational mind—Freud takes a different approach. Like Copernicus discovering that he can account for planetary orbits by making a model in which the planets go around the sun instead of the earth, Freud holds that we can understand "the will" of the individual if we make it revolve around the imagos (Freud, 1917a, p. 141). Thus, the different estimates of power or authority found in these forms of paranoia, for example, can explain how a "normal" person's ambition, or striving for perfection is to be understood. This means that complex power dynamics in society are anchored to the imagos that the child forms in psychosexual development. Although some have criticized this formulation for attributing complex intellectual powers to the infant or child, this only remains a problem so long as one views the child as atomistic. Once one views the child as primarily related, then the imagos merely conserve this relationality itself and later will be filled with content from a particular political economy.

Freud is clear that there are multiple (primary) identifications with the parents that form the superego through childhood development:

> [N]or must it be forgotten that a child has a different estimate of its parents at different periods of its life. At the time at which the Oedipus complex gives place to the super-ego they are something quite magnificent; but later they lose much of this. Identifications then come about with these later parents as well, and indeed they regularly make important contributions to the formation of character; *but in that case they only affect the ego, they no longer influence the super-ego, which has been determined by the earliest parental imagos.*
>
> *(Freud, 1933, p. 64, emphasis added; see also 1923b, pp. 31, 34, 54)*

The formation of the superego gives the individual psychological inputs for recognizing different levels of authority, class, and social power. There can be a huge difference in the felt relation that one has towards one's employer or teacher in contrast to how it feels to be introduced to a billionaire, a popular celebrity, or a leader in one's field of work or profession. From another angle, consider how it felt to be a college student and how much knowledge one attributed to one's professors and even the graduate students. Although it is common to question one's deservingness of an MA or PhD, there is some social trust in place that one's professors or others in authority must deserve to be there—someone would say something or point it out if they were not fit for the position, right? Then, in an even deeper way, consider how beyond this social trust that there is a basic trust that one will drive to work tomorrow and return home for dinner at day's end (Erikson, 1963). For some patients, this basic trust has been broken down and they live in a world in which they feel that war can break out at any moment, a demonic or ghostly force is haunting them, or a meteor could hit the earth. It is not that we are aware of the probabilities and decide what it is rational to feel or not. Instead it is whether or not our transferences to the social body or the world in general are positive or not, or caught up in psychodynamic defenses.

I do not want to stress the relation between class and transference too much, however. It is apparent that we also meet people and sometimes have a feeling that someone might be a genius, a beauty model, or some important person, without any knowledge of their actual class or status. A person may be brought up in estimation once their status is determined or they may be brought down from the ideal impression that they make on the surface. The psychoanalytic model of mind has concepts that can formalize these observations based upon different relations to the imago as the building block of the mind.[2]

As mentioned in the last quotation, the imago directly relates to the superego. Again, more precisely, when it comes to the matter of assessing authority and the perfection of other people, and measuring oneself against them, it is the ego-ideal aspect of the superego that is relevant. The ego ideal that assesses power combines with what Freud calls ego and object drives, which reference how a person can have many different motivations to relate to others or the world at large. Freud (1930) writes:

> [H]appiness, in the reduced sense in which we recognize it as possible, is a problem of the *economics of the individual's libido*. There is no golden rule which applies to everyone: every man must find out for himself in what particular fashion he can be saved. All kinds of different factors will operate to direct his choice. It is a question of how much real satisfaction he can expect to get from the external world, how far he is led to make himself independent of it, and, finally, how much strength he feels he has for altering the world to suit his wishes. In this, *his psychical constitution will play a decisive part, irrespectively of the external circumstances*. The man who is predominantly erotic will give first preference to his emotional relationships to other people; the narcissistic man, who inclines to be self-sufficient, will seek his main satisfactions in his internal mental processes; the man of action will never give up the external world on which he can try out his strength . . . success is never certain, for that depends on the convergence of many factors, perhaps on none more than on the *capacity of the psychical constitution to adapt its function to the environment* and then to exploit that environment for a yield of pleasure. A person who is born with a specially unfavourable *instinctual constitution*, and who has not properly undergone the transformation and rearrangement of his libidinal components which is indispensable for later achievements, will find it hard to obtain happiness from his external situation, especially if he is faced with tasks of some difficulty.
> *(pp. 83–84, emphasis added)*

Here Freud offers us some quick sketches of people who show stable patterns in their motivational systems. These systems are related to the general idea that people strive for happiness in different ways. For some people, their romantic life is felt to be more important than their work life, for others, time with their friends is often more important than their romantic partner. Some strive to be recognized as a top name in their field, some focus on being mediators at work and keeping harmony there, and there can be vast differences in the conscientiousness of different coworkers. As mentioned above, many only see these things as historically conditioned by certain societal discourses and deny individual psychology as having its own expressions. They take widespread cultural practices, clichés, and stereotypes about a culture and elevate them to the level of a codified human nature for a historical time period. As I slowly introduce theory throughout the chapters of this book, I will seek to show how there must be a dialectic between the individual personality and the shaping or molding that societies and families perform, and in some cases, fail to perform upon them. Children are not blank slates upon which discourse etches itself, and psychoanalysis has important implications on the sociological level. Conversely, there is cause to see that "human nature" is not ahistorical, but was likely influenced by class conflict in history.[3] It is outside of the scope of this book to go into an extended study of these important issues, but it is important to me to acknowledge them and show the prima facie connections.

II

The link between childhood development and the individual's motivational systems or "character" have been explicit in the history of psychoanalysis. To this day, even non-analysts can say that another person is anal, or mention an oral fixation, without knowing the source of these terms. However, this bodily zone relation to character often receives an exclusive focus without the references to the superego/imagos, or the sense of perfection and power that is formed in psychosexual development. In classical psychoanalysis, major figures like Ferenczi (1952), for example, relate being ambitiously driven to strive for success to childhood development:

> This almost incurable megalomania of mankind is only apparently contravened by these neurotics with whom behind the feverish search for success one at once comes across a feeling of inferiority (Adler), which is well known to the patients themselves. An analysis that reaches to the depths reveals in all such cases that these feelings of inferiority are in no sense something final, an explanation of the neurosis, but are themselves the reactions to an exaggerated feeling of omnipotence, to which such patients have become "fixed" in their early childhood, and which has made it impossible for them to adjust themselves to any subsequent renunciation. The manifest seeking for greatness that these people have, however, is only a "return of the repressed," a hopeless attempt to reach once more, by means of changing the outer world, the omnipotence that originally was enjoyed without effort.
>
> *(p. 231)*

Although the basic insight is present in this formulation, later analysts criticized this point of view by claiming it was "adultomorphic" and attributed ideas of power dynamics that are too complex for a child. However, I would argue that this is based upon these later analysts uncritically possessing an atomistic, rational chooser view of the individual. In a lot of the work of ego psychology, for example, one encounters the good, common sense view, that "values and ideals are not possible without a certain level of intellectual development" (Beres, 1958, p. 328). Granted, formulations like Ferenczi's, in the early days of analysis, do not articulate our primary relatedness in ways that are philosophically sophisticated enough, and the emphasis on primary childhood omnipotence is wrong (as I will argue later). However, what is important here is that a student of the history of psychoanalysis can see the link between childhood development, motivational systems, and character in the global sense (as opposed to minor traits).

This aspect of Freud's thought was dismissed by ego psychologists through something that appears like the conflation of thinking with *meaning* something with words. For them, the baby does not speak and the young child is not articulate, so therefore we can't ascribe values and ideals to them. Similarly, one can see the same attack made on the work of Melanie Klein, her critics claiming that she attributes too much intelligence to infants in the phantasies and internal object (imago) relations that she reports. If one views the individual as primarily separate then this view makes sense, and I would like to direct my reader to the appendix of *The Economics of Libido* (2015) for formal arguments against this common sense position. In that text, I put together Wittgenstein's private language argument and show the position he generates from his interesting philosophy of language.

Luckily, ego psychologists like Annie Reich and Edith Jacobson have kept the insight of classical psychoanalysis alive in their theoretical formulations. They attempt to make a differentiation between the ego ideal and the superego in order to satisfy the ideological influence of their time, while still recognizing the connection of childhood development on character and motivation. Despite Jacobson's lack of formalization concerning its influence, her words on the subject are quite suggestive:

> Forever close to magic imagery and yet indispensable to the ego, the ego ideal is eventually moulded from such idealized object and self images. The separate though concomitant building up of an ego ideal composed of idealized parental and self images and of realistic ego goals as well as realistic self and object representations, appears to reflect the child's simultaneous acceptance of the reality principle and his resistance to it . . . The prominent, strange, and precious quality of the ego ideal is its unreality and its distance from the real self. Although we are ordinarily perfectly aware of this, the ego ideal exerts a tremendous influence on our realistic behaviour. The vicissitudes of the ego ideal reflect, of course, the development of infantile value measures. Its deep unconscious core harbours derivatives of early notions of value, such as the idea of eternal happiness, of glamour and wealth, or physical and mental power and strength; notions which do not yet have the quality of moral ideas but, partly surviving in our ego goals, may play a paramount role in patients whose superego has never matured.
>
> *(Jacobson, 1964, pp. 110–112)*

Instead of ego and object drives that motivate the individual, Jacobson adopts the concepts of self and object representations from the ego psychology of her day. In contrast to Freud's model, which sees parental imagos form the superego through different stages of development, Jacobson, holds that the superego only becomes a fully separate system in the resolution of the phallic-Oedipus complex. For ego psychologists, this complex represents moving from dependence upon the parents to internalizing their authority and being born as a rational chooser. Seeing the superego in this way, Jacobson separates the ego ideal from it and links it to self and object representations from earlier psychosexual development. These representations stand to impede or cloud the rational individual with their unrealistic, magical ideals, or as lacunae of self-esteem, which can be represented as being injured, castrated, in danger, etc. However, Jacobson's formulations allow for the ego ideal to "exert a tremendous influence on our realistic behaviour" and her work generally points beyond the simple opposition between the phallic-oedipal superego, as a separate system, and superego precursors.

Like Jacobson, Annie Reich (1954) also has some very powerful writings on the ego ideal and its influence on our real behavior:

> It is self-evident to us that the superego identifications retain, throughout life, their special form of differentiated structures within the ego. We are used to think of earlier identifications as ego identifications; i.e., as identifications which are completely integrated into the ego, and which do not lead to a differentiation within the ego . . . [but] even early identifications do not always result in such a complete integration. Early identifications with parental qualities which are envied and admired may take place in order to undo a narcissistic hurt. They may be represented by a longing to be like the idealized parent and may lead not at all, or only in a certain degree, to a personality transformation in the desired sense. These longings must be described as ego ideals. The ego is measured against them, and self-esteem depends on the distance between them and the ego; just as, later, on the distance between ego and superego. It depends upon the level of ego development reached by a person whether or not this measuring between ego and ego ideal will result in attempts to achieve realization of these ideals. On a primitive level of ego development, such ideals may express themselves predominantly via imaginary wish fulfillment: as narcissistic fantasies. This is the more primitive method . . . of restoring injured narcissism.
>
> Narcissistic fantasies in which one sees oneself big, powerful, a genius, etc., vary in their degree of *Ichzugehörigkeit* (belonging to the ego). Sometimes they represent only a pleasurable pastime; they may, e.g., be an element of masturbation fantasies that is taken up during periods of sexual excitement. But frequently they are an essential, permanent element of the personality, against which the ego is measured. Only in this case can one consider them ego ideals.
>
> *(pp. 219–220)*

Reich, like Jacobson, also discusses attaining a true superego, in contrast to the ego ideal, and once again, we are given a sense of the ego ideal determining one's level of ambition. This time, gone are the references to the original omnipotence of the child that we see in Ferenczi, and instead, the ego is measured against the identifications with the parents and is paired with feelings of inferiority. Reich does bring up examples in which this narcissism is satisfied in fantasy or imitative behavior, which is what many later ego psychologists latch onto in her writings. However, she clearly establishes that the ego ideal translates into ambition, as seen in the quotation.

Although Reich and Jacobson are not explicit about it, the influence of the ego ideal formed in childhood still has to be balanced against other factors. For example, having very successful parents can create the sense that a child will have to do something ambitious in his or her own career pursuits without that child necessarily having a powerful, primitive ego ideal formed in psychosexual development. Similarly, ambition may be a cultural ideal in one's particular political economy and be formed as a second nature through forms of discipline and punishment.

I will give some other examples of first and second nature in the coming chapters to further illustrate this point.

Following Freud, I have no use for the concepts of self- and object representations, nor to separate the ego ideal and superego as separate systems. First, the original term of imago, which is formed after primary identification with parents or siblings is directly linked to the superego (Freud, 1933, p. 64). As I will soon show, it is possible to usurp the place of the parental imago and become one's own ideal. Freud discusses this usurpation in the psychopathology of mania (Freud, 1917d, pp. 253–255; 1921, pp. 131–133). The use of self- and object representations only serves to separate these imago relations from motivational systems. Second, Freud (1933) is explicit that the ego ideal is an aspect of his concept of the superego up to his later writings: "[w]e have allotted it the functions of self-observation, of conscience and of [maintaining] the ideal" (ibid., p. 66). It is not my intention to say that because Freud writes this, that we should unquestioningly listen to him. Rather I invoke his opinion here out of respect for the complexity of his thought and to say I think he had good reasons for it—reasons that are hinted at by his mentioning the function of self-observation first. This leads me to the third point, Freud establishes the superego as a phenomenological fact in noting that people are capable of self-observation:

> But it is more prudent to keep the agency as something independent and to suppose that conscience is one of its functions and that self-observation, which is an essential preliminary to the judging activity of conscience, is another of them. And since when we recognize that something has a separate existence we give it a name of its own, from this time forward I will describe this agency in the ego as the "*super-ego*."
>
> *(ibid., p. 60).*

This commentary from Freud's late period is just an echo of the writings of his middle period when he explicitly relates self-observation to self-consciousness, or being able to take the ego as an object. The ego ideal was introduced as part of the ego, as a

> special agency [which] is slowly formed there, which is able to stand over against the rest of the ego, which has the function of observing and criticizing the self and of exercising a censorship within the mind, and which we become aware of as our "conscience." In the pathological case of delusions of observation, this mental agency becomes isolated, dissociated from the ego, and discernible to the physician's eye. [This] fact that an agency of this kind exists, which is able to treat the rest of the ego like an object—the fact, that is, that man is capable of self-observation—renders it possible to invest [the ego with] those things which seem to self-criticism to belong to the old surmounted narcissism of earliest times.
>
> *(Freud, 1919a, p. 235; 1914a, p. 97; 1921, pp. 109–110)*

The fact that we are able to observe, criticize, and be conscious of the self is the structural function of the superego, and this can be done in moral and motivational ways. To view oneself as weak, shameful, as out of control, a loser, as weird, as presumptuous, as ugly, guilty, and to get into very early/primitive views of oneself as "a nothing," grotesque, etc., are just a few examples of the superego in action. When it is motivational and related to ideals that are supposed to make us share a sense of perfection with an imago, for example, then it is related to the ego-ideal aspect. Despite Freud's explicit formulations of self-observation and self-criticism, I have only been able to find a few analysts who represent the full import of this. "The superego," Lewis (1971) writes, "groups together all the occasions when the person is evaluating himself, either positively or negatively, and whether the context of self-evaluation is moral or nonmoral" (p. 25). Sandler (1960) and Lampl-De Groot (1947) more generally discuss self-esteem regulation and how this area is insufficiently studied. There are many more analysts who have accepted Freud's connection between the ego ideal and perfection, but these more general formulations are important because perfectionism is not the sole story of motivational self-criticism. I will show other forms of striving for happiness in the next book, but for this one I will stay with a narrow sense of perfection in order to develop a sketch of linear development.

Wealth, fame, or status are measurable in society. One's reputation has specific semiotic markers depending on how much money one makes, what degrees one has, what institutional affiliations one belongs to, what awards one has received, how much one is in the public eye, etc. Being seen by others as important, more perfect, or above them, has levels of increasing magnitude and will be the subject of Chapter 5. In parallel, the conscience aspect of the superego enters as the sense of whether others judge one as a good person. To do something unethical and be judged by, or talked about by others, as "bad," similarly has levels of greater magnitude. It is one thing to be a bad dinner guest, another to be someone with a criminal record, and still another to commit certain monstrous or heinous crimes (which have their own infamy). For the individual to be bothered by his non-ethical reputation, and the thought of his parents or their substitutes getting wind of it, is the functional definition of shame. However, the failure to live up to one's ambition directly relates to feelings of inferiority, self-hate, worthlessness, etc. that can be conceived of as motivational shame.

Freud's example of delusions of feeling like one is watched by some malevolent force, or the clinical phenomenon of depersonalization, show another aspect of the superego (Freud, 1914a, 1917c, 1921, 1933). Many patients have described depersonalization as feeling that they are not living life but watching their life as if they are in a movie. For some, this allows them to break laws and treat others badly without experiencing strong reactions of conscience. In these examples the sense of being measured in regards to one's class in society are not present, and the lack of reference to the social body goes along with the concepts of primary as opposed to secondary narcissism. I will begin to define aspects of narcissism in the next chapter, but for the moment let me point out that although the popular usage of narcissism directly references someone who measures himself as important, or as someone who should be important in the human environment, Freud's initial coinage of it is something different. Freud initially used the term to reference how "the satisfaction of the instincts is partially or totally withdrawn from the influence of other people" (Freud, 1921, p. 69). Although this may appear as if Freud is indicating an atomistic view of the individual, it still references the imagos formed in childhood development from the dependence on caregivers. Again, more will be said about this, beginning in the next chapter, but for my purposes here, this sense of satisfaction outside the influence of other people, or in seeing oneself from outside of oneself in depersonalization, are examples of primary narcissism.

There are two more important ideas that need to be mentioned here. First, not all parental and sibling imagos are felt to be perfect and superior. This relates to how there are many more motivational systems in a person than just ambition and desire for power, and concepts like the primal scene that capture a weakened image of a parent. The latter will be examined in Chapter 5, but a more formalized study of different motivational systems will be examined under the rubric of psychic bisexuality in the next book. Second, the relation to imagos is tied to the concept of id drives as the idiosyncratic forms of aggression and affection from psychosexual development (Freud, 1933, p. 120). These id drives often show up in the clinic and are directly related to anxiety states with the parental imago.[4] I will have more to say about them shortly.

In the ego and object drive model, every future relationship of the individual follows the prototype established with a parental or sibling imago in psychosexual development. The question is whether a relationship is ambivalent and based upon a specific repetition or whether it is non-ambivalent and a general repetition. For example, a relation to an authority like a teacher in school can be ambivalent and full of defiance, or the student can feel a need to ingratiate themselves to the teacher, or show some other pattern. However, not every child shows evidence of this (i.e. their relation to authority is non-ambivalent). Thus, a "narcissistic scar" or ego injury occurs after psychosexual development that sets up a repetition of an ego or object drive. This view is very close to language common to relationships: someone gets cheated on or hurt in a previous relationship and then one brings "baggage" into the new relationship. One has trust issues, jealousy, puts up "walls," or denigrates the opposite sex. In my clinical approach, it is very common for patients to return to the ego injury and get in touch with that anger. When asked where they feel the emotion in their bodies, a therapist can get all forms of idiosyncratic responses. They can feel it in their hands and want to strangle or pound the other, they can feel it in their jaw and want to bite, they can feel it in their chest, their eyes, their shoulders, their legs, etc. Discharging the anger and the idiosyncratic id drive is dynamically related to bringing "the wall" down. These idiosyncratic id drives are trans-historical and show up in myths, fables, horror movies, and stories across centuries and cultures, and are evidence of human beings sharing a common psychological foundation.

III

This now brings me to the clinical technique and the vignettes I will be sharing in this book. My training is psychoanalytic, but because I am a counselor at a community clinic, I often have to do short-term therapy with many of my patients. I do not have the luxury of simply waiting for the transference and, since many of my patients are chemically dependent, impulsive, and criminal, the stakes often feel very high. In my anxiousness about the heightened stakes, and the brevity of the time frame, I began looking into other approaches. A few years back, I began reading some Gestalt therapy books and adapted one important technique. Fritz Perls (1969) sometimes had a patient pretend to be a thing or person from a dream shared during a session, asking the patient to speak from whatever place or relation it occupied in the dream. I did not feel comfortable with asking clients to act, or pretend to be the license plate on the car in their dream, for example, and so I modified the request. I would ask patients to describe a thing or person in the dream and then see if describing a part of themselves in the same way felt true. I first tried this with a patient who repeatedly mentioned the corner ledge of a building in a dream she had shared. I asked her to use adjectives to describe the corner ledge and she said "slippery, dangerous, and cold." I was impressed by the potential anthropomorphic quality this had and when I asked her if it felt true to say this about a part of herself, as an ego statement, I was rewarded with a whole new part of her personality coming into the analysis. She told me about walking by herself at night by bars that were closing down and putting herself into very dangerous situations in which she could be assaulted, raped, or killed.

In the next few years I became more and more aware of repetitions in the clinic. Some patients keep finding abusive men or addicted romantic partners who they lie awake at night worrying about. Some will share that all their major relationships have ended because they found out that their partner cheated on them. When I got my training in EMDR, I was surprised by how well the technique worked with the superego. The practitioner elicits self-observations such as: I am powerless, I am defective, I am unsafe, I am out of control, I am undesirable, etc. in order to create a memory network of repetitions (Shapiro, 2001). One then applies bilateral stimulation (BLS) and this encourages the feelings associated with the relationships and ego injuries to surface more quickly and easily. A psychoanalyst no longer has to wait for the transference, dreams, or for slips of the tongue in order to access the repressed feelings from these ego injuries, and often the patient will produce these things sooner. However, desensitizing feelings in some of these memory networks seemed to hit a dead end. With my psychoanalytic background, I was able to see that the patient often had dynamic defenses in place that the EMDR approach does not recognize.

When I got stuck with patients I began eliciting ego and object statements in order to undo the very common defense of projective identification. Projective identification (PI) is a concept in psychoanalysis that many analysts have a hard time defining and that is used differently by different schools. The use I give it is based upon Melanie Klein's original use of it, as an operation in which both the bad and hated parts of the self, and potentially some of the good parts too, are projected into other people (Klein, 1975, p. 8). In effect, the person reverses the relation between himself and the parental imago (internal object), so that he acts the part of a parental-substitute to someone who represents the self imago (with its ambivalent relation to the parental imago).[5] Undoing this defense allowed for the creation of a new memory network and permitted the work to continue. However, after this insight, I began to see there were many opportunities to begin memory networks from the current repetitions in a patient's life. Let me give a couple examples from my practice:

> Client has recently got his sex drive back after previously saying he has no desire for a romantic relationship. Strong themes of wanting to feel desired and attractive have begun to come into the analysis. However, in today's session he comes in with a complaint that there is a woman he is attracted to at his work and that he realizes that he "act[s] different" once he is attracted to someone. He says he "freeze[s] up" and acts like he doesn't like them. I ask him to focus on the woman he mentioned specifically and to tell me what she might think about him or how he acts around her. He says that she might think he has "a bad vibe," is "too good," "stuck up," "uninterested," and that she might feel "rejected" and feel "frustrated or angry" with him. I ask him to put these into ego and object statements about someone from his past (i.e. "You have a bad vibe, you think you are too good, you are stuck up, you are uninterested in me, and I feel rejected, and frustrated and angry with you"), and to say them in his head, and see who comes to mind. He mentions an ex-girlfriend, his "dad," a group of friends from when he was a teenager, and after a longer pause adds his mother. I ask him to start with the most recent one and ask him to picture whatever moments with her come to

mind and see which one is the strongest and I begin BLS. He tells me about a time that his ex and another man seemed to be texting while in the same room with him while a couple other people were "hanging out and getting high." He suspected that they were having an affair but had no solid proof until after. He emphasizes how "disrespectful" they were being and his tone is incredulous and sarcastic as he describes the details of the memory. I ask him to stay with the memory and he tells me that he can feel it in his chest after resuming BLS. I ask him to see if it wants to grow, move, or develop and resume BLS. He tells me that it grew in his chest and he feels a lot of anger start to come in. I ask him if he feels the anger in his chest or if there's another place in his body that he feels power in, or from where he'd like to express his anger. He tells me that he feels it in his hands and I ask him to see how it would like to come out and resume BLS. He tells me that he can picture wrapping his hands around someone's neck and "choking the shit out of them." I ask him to picture the memory with his ex and the other man and to start with his words and tell them what he didn't say and told me (i.e. how "disrespectful" they were being). I tell him that if he still feels anger after the words that he should let his body express whatever physical urge he still feels, so that the anger can be discharged. I resume BLS and I can see the intensity of client's anger in his eyes as he's discharging it in his mind's eye. After he signals me to stop, he tells me that he "killed both of them" and then traces how he yelled at them at first and then had "ripped the phone out of her hand and smashed her in the face with it." He says that she "begged me not to kill [the man]" and "tried to stand up for him" and so after choking him to death, he returned to do the same to her. I ask him how he feels and he says that this was "uncomfortable for sure" but that he also feels "more alive." As is usual, the discharge of anger often allows for the inferiority or self-criticism to come up. Client begins to talk about how he felt like the other man was "above [him]" and "too good . . . like her." I interpret, "Like they are the adults and you're just a kid?" and he eagerly agrees and then adds that he feels like he's "always missing something in life. . .in the conversation, like there's a secret behind [his] back." He then brings up the memory of hanging out with his friends as teenagers and how they'd be talking and he felt like he was "missing something."

Another client discloses a "random hookup" with a "girl" he contacted on the Internet. I explore this with him and it becomes apparent that he has a history of "ghosting" women (i.e. that he would sleep with and then disappear and not answer their calls or texts). Client shows a little defensiveness as he talks about these women, even though I don't feel like I'm being judgmental at all. I agree with him as he talks about how they are adults and know that this is about sex and that they can't have too much by way of expectations. However, as he gets into one specific woman, who he had slept with a few times and who liked his artwork, I ask him if she might have had some expectations. He affirms that it was likely and I ask him to guess

> what she might have thought about him. He says that she might think he is "interesting," that he is "magical," and that she'd "like to be close to [him]." I ask him what she might think about him when he disappears and he adds that she might "worry that [he's] dead." I ask him to say these as (ego and object) statements about someone from his past: "You are interesting, you are magical, I'd like to be close to you, but you are gone and I'm worried you are dead." He tells me that his mother comes to mind. She was an addict and he recounts how she would show up for a couple months at his grandparents' house, with whom he lived when he was younger, and she would "do good" for a while and then end up disappearing.

In this last vignette, my patient has taken on the role of the parental imago; the anxiety and fear that he had with his mother is projected into the women that he "ghosts." This is a common theme in many of the addicted patients with whom I work. They may have a loving romantic partner or family member, yet they will disappear and often put themselves in dangerous situations that cause those who care for them to worry and lose sleep. Such patients behave like they have no fear or anxiety, while the romantic partner or family member is full of anxiety and often works hard to get the addict help, of which they seldom make use. In *The Economics of Libido* (2015), I argue that the two deep objects of psychoanalysis are perfection and death. Both are negative qualities: neither can be known directly by finite beings and their very existence can be understood as a negation of the finite.[6] Thus, not only is there the more perfect other, who is above you and makes you feel inferior, there is also the dead other, who is interesting, good hearted, or bright, but who leaves, disappears, or dies. The dead other can register as outside of life, but in higher levels of development it can register as outside of the social body through being ignored, marginalized, and not having what it is "normal" to have. In the first clinical example above, my patient was similarly in PI, but in a way that registers superiority and power more than the sense of being close to someone who feels interesting, exciting, or authentic. However, in both examples, there is a sense of one person being the child and one being the parent or parental-substitute.

Like the above example of death, "omnipotence" or grandiosity similarly belongs to the parental imago of perfection and is not the natural state of the infant or child. Here is another example of using ego and object statements to undo the usurpation of the parental imago of perfection in PI:

> Client is experiencing a block in a memory we are focusing on. He is having difficulty accessing the feelings and says that he feels itchy. I get him to stay with this itchy sensation and resume BLS. When we stop, he describes it as staying about the same and not developing in any way. I ask him what words he'd use to describe it and he says, "little, annoying, and irritating." I ask him what comes to mind if he says these as object statements. He says a bug, and then a fly. I then ask him if any people come to mind with the same object statements and with the added idea of them "bugging him." He brings up some

co-workers who annoyed him in the past and pairs it with his "snarky side." I ask him to be more specific, and he shares about someone on his crew who was an "older guy, not on his game, not up to standards." He adds, that this guy on his crew would "slow everyone down, was annoying, not efficient, and holding everyone back." Client explains that his snarkiness is expressed as teasing. He says that this teasing "was fun" and that it "pushed people to do better." I ask client to guess at what this specific crew member might think about him and his "fun." Client says that this coworker would probably "feel like an idiot" and would think client was "a know it all." We run out of time for this session.

Next session client denies any explicit processing. However, he tells me that he's reading a book on Vikings and how he likes warriors, but needs the subject matter to be partly true or historical—he doesn't "go in for fantasy and dragons." I ask him what attracts him to Vikings and not other warrior groups, and he tells me about how they didn't have a king and that they were closer to anarchists and had a "group mentality" that he liked. I get him to unpack this a bit and he tells me that he's against big government and dictators and adds with uncharacteristic flamboyance that he "can't follow a king." He goes on to say that when he thinks about dictators that "crazies, and Hitlers" come to mind. I ask him how these kings and dictators would think about those they "rule." He says that such a man would see others as "weaker, below him, his opinion counts and theirs don't . . . they can't say a lot." In contrast, in a smaller government, where people who have a group mentality lead, client says that the leader is "worried about their well-being, is not all about power, and is open to other ideas." This leader doesn't think: "this is the way it is, and it's not up for discussion." Client seems more animated than usual when he's talking about these things. I take the object statements from the king/dictator and ask client to say them and see if they feel true to say about anyone (instead of eliciting the ego statements of superiority, which might be harder for him to own). He tells me that his children come up, but quickly rationalizes how one has to be this way with kids. I go along with his thoughts on children, but then ask him if the statements might feel right with anyone else, and to say them again in his head. He tells me that some people from his work crew come to mind. He then rationalizes that it's not about him or the work crew, but about getting the job done. I counter that "Hitlers" might say it's not about them but about the glory of the motherland. He smiles and agrees with this, and I point out that he obviously has a good work ethic, but that these healthy things in him don't need therapy, they are healthy. I ask him to focus on whether there is a small part of him that identifies with the king-dictator and he agrees to and we begin BLS. He tells me that it does feel right and that this part of him comes out at work too. I ask him to focus on it and resume BLS. He reports that he feels it in his chest and back. I ask him to see if the sensation in these zones wants to grow bigger or move to somewhere else. He surprises me and adds with remorse that he "rides his son sometimes" and that he "nitpicks him more

> than others." He says that he feels "disappointed with [himself] for doing it to him." Client added that this is "more of [his] father coming out." I ask him to focus on when his father made him feel like he was weaker and like his opinion didn't count" and resume BLS. He brings up a couple memories.

While grandiosity may be easier to pinpoint in lower-functioning patients, such identifications occur across the spectrum with varying degrees of subtlety. In the example above, my patient's snarkiness and disposition to "type A" micro-management with others is such an expression, but his associations to Hitlers, kings, and tyrants illustrates the connection of his personality type to the grandiosity of the parental imago. His ability to accept this connection allowed for a reversal, and he began to consciously identify with his son and coworker because he had felt that way in his earlier relationship to his father. This reversal, and the consequent softening of the patient's character, illustrates how grandiosity is not primary. In my clinical experience, omnipotence is always defensive and can be reversed. Most of the time the patient will recall childhood memories of mistreatment from parents or parental-substitutes, but sometimes PI arises as a defense against one's own transgressions against the parental imago. I will turn to the conscience aspect of the superego, and how it can be the basis of defense shortly.

In addition to EMDR, sensorimotor psychotherapy (Ogden, Minton, & Pain, 2006) has provided a useful direction for research. While EMDR focuses on the negative cognitions (or critical superego self-observations), elicits a memory network, and then checks them against opposite positive cognitions, the sensorimotor approach focuses more on the uncompleted action in the body. Tracking non-verbals and asking patients to lift up their shoulders, narrow their eyes, or fold their arms in exaggeration of these micro-gestures can often get into important memories or feeling states. In line with my psychoanalytic knowledge, I consider the expression of the id drive, which is caught up with the hatred or anger of the ego injury, to be more important than the overly cognitive instillation of a positive self-observation. With this perspective in mind, I began to have patients return themselves to the memories in which the ego injuries occurred, and instead of suppressing their anger and id drives, I asked them to express those emotions, drives, and resulting actions in their mind's eye. As seen in the example of the double murder by strangulation above, all manner of classical sadism and even some new forms that I had never read about in the literature began to show up. Patients would shoot laser beams out of their eyes and disintegrate others, take pins and poke holes in others so that they deflated and became "skin sacks," terrify others with the immensity of their power and size until the others became puddles on the ground, break their jaws, peel off their skin, and many more.

I am sure at this point that there is a reader who must be thinking that this does not sound therapeutic and, moreover, that I might be encouraging psychopathy. Perhaps there is a reader with a subtler thought, about how the *verbalization* of this aggression is what is important, and that by having patients express it in their mind's eye, I am neglecting the consolidation of their ego strength. To the first, let me say that there is a lifetime between thought and expression. Far from seeing patients becoming psychopaths, the discharge of the suppressed impulses in their mind's eye processes aggression. Destructiveness, which would otherwise remain repressed and contribute towards their self-destructive behavior or future acts of destruction towards others, is let go. The therapeutic benefit is apparent in the here and now; it is evident in the release of chronic muscular tensions, which previously held the activated id impulses in place, for example. The unwinding of a face twisted in resentment, or hearing a patient talk about the warmth, wholeness, or well-being that enters after the aggression has been imagined and then discharged, often translates into the patient distancing herself from bad relationships and reporting new, healthier relationships or goals. A person who is less divided, less conflicted, and more at ease with themselves, will be less of a danger to others, not more. To the person arguing for the importance of verbalizing and the primacy of speech, I would only say that much of this work is done with an intrapsychic conflict model in mind. This doesn't mean that I don't recognize the importance of a deficit model, and in Chapters 5 and 6 I will show that the full internalization of the imago has an important place in Freud's model of the personality. Ultimately, I would say that the burden of proof lies at the feet of those who claim a deficit issue is at stake in the verbalization of aggression. They should be able to provide proof of the cognitive limits in their patients, and moreover, that the individual has always had such a limitation. This should be a simple quantitative claim to research.

Along with these criticisms, I also expect others to tell me that expression of feelings and impulses in the mind's eye is simply fantasy or make-believe and thus cannot be beneficial. My first response is that clinicians should be focused on outcomes and that they should see for themselves whether this approach results in the patient overcoming the relationship pattern or the psychopathology involved. Second, if such critics want to ignore the somatic changes that patients will express in this work, and the psyche–soma parallelism that is indicated in psychoanalytic theory, then they are in the same position in which they see me. They are left with a model in which the patient has repressed a feeling, a perception, or an idea, and that this is similarly "all in her head." If the patient expresses the repressed feeling in her mind's eye, then this is analogous to however she defended against it "in her head," through the act of repression. I understand that higher-functioning adults spend most of their time oriented to their goals, duties, and responsibilities and that acts of fantasying and imagination can seem childish. However, one cannot claim that their orientation is evidenced as primary in childhood development. Autistic children who do not go on to learn language, and are left in this state of dependency, illustrate that more abstract cognitive functions are primary (Tustin, 1988a, 1988b). Interactions with others, measuring oneself in relation to them, and goal directed behavior is a later development.

When one considers the helplessness and dependency of the infant, there are inborn instincts like sucking at the breast or grasping with the hand, but the early ego drives are something different. These ego drives were dubbed epistemophilic drives by classical analysts, and are underpinned by relation to the parental imagos and are functions that can be caught up in psychopathology.[7] The early ego drives push the child to give his attention to new things and paths, and to want to take things apart and figure out how they work or are put together in the external world. They also drive the child to form connections between things in his internal world that aren't simply empirically given, to interact with the sensuousness of an object's physical form (physiognomy) in acts of mimicry, and to express feeling through the sensuousness of the arts. The primacy of play for young children should show the enormity of the internal world, the early stages of development, and the importance of acts of fantasying. The practical and often compulsive pursuits of many adults later in life does not prove the unimportance of fantasying and play. Instead, it only shows how pervasive psychopathology and early stage defenses are for many people. This has led many to observe "the depressing contrast between the radiant intelligence of a healthy child and the feeble intellectual powers of the average adult" (Freud, 1927, p. 47). How many adults read their last book in high school? How many of those who have continued reading, have only become better at rationalizing the views and dogmas with which they already identified?

Returning to clinical technique, those with worries regarding the emphasis on the aggressive and ugly side of this work, should know that the violent dramas in the mind's eye soon led to moral encounters. Going back to ego injuries, these often bring up shame, remorse, and bad conscience as that which overstimulates and becomes repressed, in contrast to hate, for example. Here is another vignette:

> Client is with a woman who has severe mental health issues and who has done very hurtful things to him (physical abuse, cheating, stealing money for drugs, etc.). He can express that a part of him feels like he should leave her, but also tells me that a part of him doesn't want to. He reports that his girlfriend can also say horribly mean things to him in her fits of rage, and client feels like he's begun to "hysterically" adopt her anxiety. He says that he can feel himself fighting not to mirror her fits of rage, when he is arguing with her, and notices how he gets anxiety in situations in which he has seen her have anxiety. In session with him, I tell him that it seems like he is adopting the bad traits that afflict her, and I ask him if it feels like he's trying to help her in some way by doing so? Despite my failure to articulate this well, client agrees enthusiastically with what I said, and adds that "she doesn't see how much [he does] for her." I ask him to complete the sentence: "If she could see how much I took on her pains and problems then she might." He says, "care more, not take me for granted, not be so selfish or spoiled." I ask him to put these into ego and object statements and to tell me who comes to mind from his past (i.e. "I should care more, I took you for granted, I've been selfish and spoiled, I don't see how much you've done for me). Client says that his family comes to mind, and he names a few relatives. I ask him to focus on who sticks out the most and he quickly says that his grandmother does. He says that "she's stuck by [his] side [his] whole life" and "she gave [him] chance after chance and went above and beyond." "I slapped her in the face," he adds, figuratively.

> I ask him to picture her in his mind's eye how she would be looking upon him, if she were to see him again. He says that she looks perfect and that she's smiling and he begins crying. I ask him to continue picturing her and to articulate the remorse he just told me about, and to express it to her. I begin BLS, and he does so. When he signals me to stop the BLS, he tells me that she now looks angry and disappointed with him. He brings up the last time he talked to her and how she hung up the phone on him. I ask him if it feels true if he says "I deserve to be cut off," and he says it does. He then adds that he pushed her to the point that she had to cut him off. He then adds that he's not talking to his child or his family. I interpret that he's treating them like his grandmother started to treat him, and that he's replaying how his grandmother felt towards him before with how he feels towards his girlfriend. He looks lost in thought, like there is some processing going on, and I ask him to try to talk to the representation of his grandmother again, really let her understand how he feels, and then give an apology. I begin BLS and after a minute or so he stops following my fingers and says that she forgives him and she loves him with tears coming down his cheeks. I ask him to scan his body to see if he's holding on to anything else. He says that his heart feels different and so does his breath. He says he feels excitement and love but is also just serene.

In this example, my patient projectively identified with his girlfriend. The way he saw her, was the way he had been with his grandmother. He pushed his grandmother too far, she cut him off, and he received an ego injury from this.[8] It is possible that he could have continued to find a new parental-substitute from whom he could take "too much," as he did with his grandmother, but instead he defended against this repetition. He usurped the position of the parental imago and found someone to play the self imago. This relation to his grandmother did not prove to be the only factor that determined his object-choice (the desire to be with his girlfriend) and it is important to see that there is a confluence of several determinants in such relations. With some patients, I am much more explicit with asking them to make an apology. I explain to them that it is not about the other person so much as whether they believe themselves. If they truly know that they would not do something again, then they can forgive themselves through the internal representation of the imago. Some patients tell me that the representation of the wronged person does not forgive them. This can go along with admissions that stopping the offending behavior may be beyond their capabilities at present, come from defenses that suppress a full apology, or link the transgression to an earlier relation. Additionally, many patients need to express disappointment in and criticism of parents or parental-substitutes, and in picturing this in their mind's eye, the struggle is with the imago accepting accountability for what he or she had done. There will be some examples of this, and variations of technique in later chapters.

Psychoanalytic knowledge also provided the base for another development in clinical technique.

Often times while using BLS, one gets to the point where the patient is aware of sensations, often tension, in a certain bodily zone (the hands, the chest, the stomach, the diaphragm, the face, etc.). Eigen (1977), the great phenomenologist of psychoanalysis, observes that "feelings of power and energy rise and fall and become concentrated in specific bodily zones as well as remain unpredictably fluid" (p. 36) "The person first experiences a defensive consciousness in relation to the rise of bodily feeling," he writes, "[t]he ego is interested in, stimulated and frightened by the unanticipated world of continuous and varied body sensation and feelings it begins to glimpse" (ibid.) In traditional EMDR, one simply asks patients to notice it and continue the BLS, which can sometimes go nowhere and be exhausting. Sometimes, using sensorimotor techniques, the patient might have a sense for what is being held in the tension, or a sense for how his or her body wants to express the tension itself, but sometimes this too goes nowhere. At one point, I got the impression from a patient that there was a strongly felt sense of an internal image that went beyond the sensations he felt in his body. Here is an example of how patients can hint or suggest this process on their own:

> Client talks about being a good person who has "faith in others" and is "hopeful." He adds that he has "positive energy" and that others "latch on to him": both other good people and "users." Users want his help, see that they can gain from him, and hope to get "extra" from him. I tell him that it sounds like he has a surplus of energy, money, or positivity to spare in his life and people see that in him, but I then ask if he ever gets or feels depleted. He says he can feel "burnt out, like he's run thin, frustrated, disappointed, and not feel appreciated." He spontaneously tells me that he is one of the only employees that comes in to work on his own time and that he does a lot extra for his boss. Then he tells me how his boss recently wanted him to come in for more extra hours that he wouldn't be paid for and that he was pretty frustrated by this. I begin BLS after I hear the anger in his voice about this, and I ask him to feel his bodily response. He says that he feels it in his chest and the anger is growing.
>
> I tell him to picture his boss in his mind's eye and say all the things he wants to without holding back. I ask him to speak from the anger in his chest, but to also see if his body needs to physically express itself. We begin BLS and when he signals me to stop, he reports that the representation of his boss looked disappointed after he did this.
>
> I ask him to put together the implicit thoughts of the boss's feelings towards him and client says that his boss is "disappointed" in him, that client "used to go that extra mile," and that he "used to be better." I ask him to turn these into ego and object statements ("I am disappointed in you, you used to go that extra mile and now you don't, you used to be better") and see if anyone from his past shows up. Client says an ex-girlfriend comes up. He explains how she had "invested more" and had went "that extra mile" in the first six months of the relationship, but that she then didn't give as much. I ask him to focus on the

> time that he saw this in her and felt disappointed, and begin BLS. Client says that he feels it again in his chest, but also in his jaw. I ask him to alternate his attention between both and see which one is bigger or gets more of his focus, and resume BLS. Client reports that the sensation in his jaw had grown and seems more important to him. He mentions that it feels like he "can't move his jaw" and "it's like it's made of stone." I ask him to take this internal felt sense and say how it might look externally, if a person looked on the outside like he felt inside. He begins describing a man with "sunken eyes" who looks "sad." He says that this man literally "looks like a picture" and is "totally still." Client interestingly adds that he "doesn't expect him [this stone man] to move." Because of the negation, I ask client to "fast forward" this image of the man five minutes, then five days, then five years, and ask him what he pictures happening to this man in the future. After an answer of nothing at the five-year mark, I ask client to see if there is any sense of the effect that time might have on him or whether the man is outside of time. Client then says that he pictures the man slowly "disintegrating": starting "from his head down." He says the stone man would just be "blown to dust in a gentle breeze." I ask him to picture the dust into which the man disintegrated, and to see if it feels right to picture this in his chest. Client agrees and I begin BLS. His face soon turns red, seemingly in embarrassment that it feels right to picture it. I tell him to let the sensations in his chest fully map on to the picture and to let me know when the process is complete. When client signals that it is, I ask him to tell me how it felt right. He says that it felt right in his heart and that he pictured his heart turning to dust and being blown by the wind until it was fully "disintegrated." However, he then adds that in its place, the picture of a full, new heart emerged. I ask him to focus on this new heart and to see if the rest of his body has any reaction to it—if it wants to somehow change how the rest of his body feels. I resume BLS and after he signals me to stop, he tells me that the tension in his jaw and chest are gone and he feels like he can move his tongue too. He says that he felt tension in his hands go away as well. I ask him if it feels like there might still be more change or development and we quickly resume BLS for a few moments, but then tells me that it doesn't feel like anything wants to change or develop further. I ask him to float back to another time he felt like this in his life and install the memory of well-being to which he associates. We then return to the memory of his ex.

Whenever a patient is stuck in sensation, I will ask something along the lines of: "if someone, or some thing, looked on the outside like it feels inside your [chest, shoulders, stomach, etc.], what do you picture?" Patients will have an answer almost every time, and they will be able to tell me almost instantly if it feels right to introject the picture that they project out. As seen in the example above, sometimes there is an intensity described in the picture or the patient will say something about it in a negation (i.e. "I don't think he [the projected person] is angry"). Both of these examples show the potential of the image or symbol to change. I remember one client who pictured the face of a green goblin and described how it had a long nose and a metal sheet that was worn on top of its head like some kind of hat. Because there was something covered up (visual negation) I asked him what the goblin might look like without the metal hat. He told me that under the hat he pictured neither hair, scalp, nor bone, but an exposed brain. It was this brain that he was able to introject into his own head to move things forward. After patients tell me that it feels right to picture the image inside of them, or that they can feel how some part of their body wants to move or look like the introjected image, I ask them to let it map on to their sensations. Once I verify with the patient that the image is fully embedded, I ask them if their body around the zone reacts to having the picture inside or if their mind reacts with a memory, a thought about when this came into them, who it was with, or if it produces a feeling. These introjections can sometimes appear to be ends in themselves. Tension in the area is processed or, as in the example above, a damaged or corrupted symbol is replaced with a new one. However, most of the time I consider this aspect of the work as a way of temporarily getting around a "block." What is central is that one returns to the memory that was initially blocked. Usually the patient is able to get into the feeling that could not be fully accessed in previous attempts, and this allows us to continue through the original memory network.[9]

The salience of projecting out images and symbols, and introjecting them, came from the importance of pre-verbal cognition in psychoanalytic thought. For example, Ferenczi (1952) discusses how symbols are underwritten by a mimetic relation in which the child "learns to represent by means of his body the whole multifariousness of the outer world" (p. 228). This means that a person can "feel" his or her way into the form of both human and non-human objects and things. A weeping willow tree, for example, can remind one of the shape of a human body that is downcast in sadness. A tree with sharp angles and a gnarled form can produce a feeling of evil or fear. We feel into forms, and although the mimetic sense varies from person to person, there is ample evidence for its existence. Eigen (2016) is careful to make sure psychoanalysts do not regard images as second-class citizens and that all the "inner states and tendencies" that expressive language can transmit "can happen with images of sound, as well as sight" (p. 616).

The post-modern influence on psychoanalysis has left these insights to rot in favor of semiotics and social constructivism, but Freud clearly saw the importance of preverbal cognition. Despite the importance of language in the talking cure, Freud (1915b) is unequivocal that "the system *Ucs.* contains the thing-cathexes of the objects, the first and true object-cathexes" (p. 201). He also gives this formulation again when he writes about melancholia:

> In melancholia, accordingly, countless separate struggles are carried on over the object, in which hate and love contend with each other; the one seeks to detach the libido from the object, the other to maintain this position of the libido against the assault. The location of these separate struggles cannot be assigned to any system but the *Ucs.*, the region of the memory-traces of *things* (as contrasted with *word*-cathexes).
>
> *(Freud, 1917d, pp. 256–257)*

The unconscious is comprised of thing-presentations that relate to the parental and sibling imagos that make up the superego. Our feelings towards our parents, siblings, and their substitutes can become ambivalent to such a degree that the feelings can reach an intensity that forces them to become repressed. Similarly, a disappointment with a love object can be so sudden that its intensity becomes overwhelming. This overstimulation will lead to anxiety and

> when once a state of anxiety establishes itself, the anxiety swallows up all other feelings; with the progress of repression, and the more those ideas which are charged with affect and which have been conscious move down into the unconscious, all affects are capable of being changed into anxiety.
>
> *(Freud, 1909a, p. 270)*

Again, this process will occur whenever one's drives encounter external or internal opposition to expression, and become overstimulating, or when feelings are too sudden and strong. It can occur with social humiliations, fear that one's reactions would put one in jail and cause shame, or because one's pride does not allow one to express a feeling, for example. The resulting ego injury from the mortification, anger, or abandonment reaction will result in an ego defense. Depending on the individual's economics of libido, this can mean an ego defense at the phallic stage or at an earlier stage.[10] The central type of example Freud (1917d) gives of this is in melancholia, in which a jilted lover introjects her angry, debased view of the beloved and begins to self-revile herself in a way that he or she would have reviled the lover. As mentioned above, it is also common that instead of this kind of defense, the ego injury itself is what is repeated or transferred to new objects. A bad imago will be created and it will be transferred to every new relationship in either her love life, work life, or in her friendships, or cause ambivalence with the parent or sibling who was the prototype of the relation.

The importance of parapraxis and language for Freud, is that the ego injuries that become repressed, are in a state without words, and some part of the mind is drawn to fill in the blank. He writes:

> Now, too, we are in a position to state precisely what it is that repression denies to the rejected presentation in the transference neuroses: what it denies to the presentation is translation into words which shall remain attached to the object. A presentation which is not put into words, or a psychical act which is not hyper-cathected [by words], remains thereafter in the *Ucs.* in a state of repression.
>
> *(Freud 1915b, p. 202)*

Associations in dreams, slips of the tongue, etc., can get us back to the repressed ego injury and imago, or the activated id drive. However, the other aspect of the thing-presentation (the imago), is the mimetic, pre-verbal thinking that relates to it and id drives. In the above clinical example, we have a bodily zone, the chest, and the idea of the heart being disintegrated. Although there was an ego injury that caused my patient to experience a part of himself as disintegrated, I did not work with the imago and the id drive (to disintegrate) but with the image of the zone. This bodily zone gave the mimetic sense of the stone man, with sunken eyes, who looked sad, and in applying the state of disintegration to himself, the patient was able to undo the self-observation of the part of himself that was destroyed.

There can be no doubt that the body provides both the basis upon which symbols are created and provides the link between cultures separated both geographically and temporally.[11] With this dimension re-opened in psychoanalytic practice, the great promise of psychoanalysis, to unriddle form and metaphor in the arts can begin again. However, the link between an image, bodily zone, and a specific imago from childhood development are hardly explicit in the clinical technique. What is going to be more valuable are the artistic representations that also show the level of authority in question. With enough data, the symbols can be correlated to both childhood development and the specific motivational systems of psychic bisexuality. I hope to show the way forward in this realm in the next book.

Upon reflection, it does not seem right to imply that psychoanalysis is the only intellectual home for ideas about mimesis or pre-verbal cognition. Although it recognizes those things, they are not particularly emphasized or made much of in the classical literature. However, it is fair to say that without psychoanalysis, I would not have recognized the importance of symbols and images in relation to particular bodily zones. The introjection of an image might make sense to a non-analyst, if it concerns the physical comportment and/or physiognomy of another human. However, in psychoanalysis psyche–soma parallelism suggests that the body can be broken down, displaced, condensed, etc. as much as the mind can be. In doing this work, I have had people introject colors and whiteness, sounds, images of musculature without skin, different feelings of heat and coldness, black holes and nothingness (absences), fire, electricity, geometric shapes, rain and clouds, landscapes, and more. I will not be able to formalize these ideas until the next book, but I would like to leave my reader with something unquestionably psychoanalytic.

One of the surprises in using this technique is how often one comes across breast and phallic symbols. The principle of assessing this is very simple. Often something spherical like a balloon, planet, apple, ball, etc., resembles a breast and is destroyed in the projection. These forms of destruction often relate to the ways in which Klein (1932, 1975) writes about the breast being sucked dry, torn into bits and pieces, etc. Similarly, objects that are long and thin like arrows, bananas, flagpoles, long noodles, and untied coat hangers are phallic objects. It is often not the breast or phallus that is internalized but the destroyed breast or phallus. Here's an example:

> I have done assertiveness work with client and he reports that several people in his life have been "shocked" with him and how he's been able to say no. I ask him what else is going on in his life, and he excitedly tells me he watched *The Goonies* the other day, and about how he loves the character Data. This

develops into a theme of how client identifies as the person in his friend group who has to have crazy ideas, music, or something to offer the others. As we explore further, he begins to express how he's not a full member of the friend group, but more of a cartoon character of sorts that they put up with. He can't just be there and be a "person," and has to do something to deserve to belong. However, as we go further into this theme, he brings up a friend, his "best friend," who has no job, plays video games all the time, and would just be alone if it wasn't for him. I ask him what he thinks would happen to his friend, if client was no longer in his life? Client says that his friend would "disappear and go off the grid." Client goes into how he's "the charismatic one," and his friend is the asocial one, and gets into some more particulars of the relationship. Afterwards, I ask client how much this resembles the relationship with his mother (who he had previously referred to as having been his best friend) and if he was the asocial one with her? He says that she "tried to make him the asocial one" but that he would talk and say things "with no filter" and that she'd often "get butt hurt about it." He pauses strangely, and then suddenly adds, "I talk too much" and "I need to shut up." I ask him to focus on this feeling and begin BLS. He registers it in his heart. I ask him to stay with the feeling and to see if it wants to develop (get bigger, move, get smaller) and continue the BLS. He feels like it is the same, so I ask him to project it out. He says that he sees a balloon on a bed of nails. I ask him to explain and he says that a balloon on a nail will pop it but when it is "10 nails" then it evens out the pressure and it doesn't pop. I ask him to pay attention to this set up and whether he pictures the balloon just staying there, resting on the nails, or if anything eventually happens. He thinks for a few moments, and then theatrically slams his hand down on the desk, signaling that the balloon will be popped. I ask him where his attention goes, to the bed of nails or to the leftovers of the balloon. He says to the latter and I ask him to picture the deflated remnants and to see whether they feel right to introject into his heart or chest. After I resume BLS, he signals that it feels right and that it fully embeds there. Then he tells me that the deflated balloon slowly begins stretching across his chest. I tell him to follow the process to completion and he does.

I ask him what this stretched balloon feels like and he tells me that it reminds him of when he "gets in trouble" and how his "heart beats really hard." He also tells me that when he talks with "no filter" that it's a rush too, and "maybe even talking in general is a rush." We discuss the asocial side of him and how he used to be quiet, but he feared "becoming invisible." He adds that "being center of attention is cool," but that part of the issue is that he "doesn't like the quiet." He suddenly switches gears and renames his asocial side his "timid" side and talks about how as a kid that "even [his] birthdays were never about [him]." He says that his parents invited over their friends and they all got drunk. However, he adds that his parents' friends were also his friends and that he didn't have any friends his age. After

> saying this, and seemingly recognizing how alone he was as a child, he stares blankly and begins giving off poetic phrases, like "I don't like living behind a curtain." This ends with client saying that he "doubt[s] that anyone wants to talk to [him]; [he] just talks to talk." In the self-pity of his loneliness, I ask him to focus on this feeling and resume BLS. He reports that his stomach feels "empty." I continue the BLS and he says that it is also a little painful and squeamish. I ask him to imagine that someone sees him from the outside and how they might imagine he looks and he says "sad" (with nothing else coming to mind). I ask him to put these into object statements and he says that his grandpa comes to mind. He tells me about how his grandpa is alone, and no one visits him, and that it's "sad." I ask him to picture his grandpa looking this way and to see if a reaction shows up in his body, and resume BLS. He does so and says that it now feels like "shit/garbage" in his stomach. I ask him to stay with this feeling and see if it wants to develop. During BLS, he tells me that it doesn't want to develop, so I ask him to project it out. He tells me that it looks like "an asshole who is pissed off and screaming." I repeat asshole? He asks me if I know Alex Jones and explains how he has a red face and begins to do an impression of him saying that "the tap water is making the friggin' frogs gay." I ask him to introject this image in and to see if it feels right. He says that it does and emphasizes that the sensations map on strongly in his jaw, and I continue the BLS. He tells me his jaw "is straining super hard" and he opens it and massages it a little. I ask him to stop moving it and to just to let "the asshole" fully embed. He goes along with this and eventually signals that it is in. Then I ask him how his body is reacting to it, now that it's in. He tells me that it's being dissolved. I continue the BLS and he then signals that it's done. I ask him if there is any sense of well-being or relief in his jaw and he says yes and I ask him when he's felt like this in his past. He says in high school when he felt like his opinion counted and he was listened to. He tells me that having his opinion valued even though he didn't have a BA was a big deal. I ask him to let the memory soak in and anchor it. We then return to the picture of the loneliness of his grandpa.

Introjecting the deflated remnants of the breast symbol helped this patient to access a previously undisclosed part of his personality. As noted in his inability to say no to others, his economics of libido is on the passive pole of personality development. His feelings of aloneness had triggered a reaction formation of him "talking like an asshole" on his active pole, in order to fill up the silence. This work with images allowed the reaction formation to be dissolved once his PI with his grandpa's social death, was undone. However, as indicated, my patient still had to return to the ego injury caused by his compassion for his grandpa, and this brought him to earlier repetitions concerning his feelings of pity.

Just as the imagos of perfection and death arise from the negation of the finite, I understand the phallus arises as a symbol from the negation of the breast. As Klein (1932) observes, there is an underlying "equation of the breast with the penis" (pp. 213–214). "[T]he frustration [one] has suffered from [the] mother's breast," she writes, "creates in [one] an imaginary picture of [the] father's penis as an organ which, unlike the breast, can provide [one] with a tremendous and never-ending oral gratification" (ibid., p. 271). To see the phallus as the negation of the frustrating breast gets rid of any sense of it having some innate or essential superiority. I understand that my reader might have worries about me sneaking in ideas that legitimize the patriarchy, "phallocentrism," or the superiority of men, but I would like to ask for some patience. The clinical technique produces many breast and phallic symbols and they are in need of an explanation.

This work with symbols has progressed in a few ways, as has the work with ego and object statements. Regarding the latter, I will give examples in the following chapters that showcase how intrapsychic symptoms and conflicts originate from interpsychic ego injuries. Regarding the former, I have become much more sensitive to the metaphorical language that patients use to describe emotional states or interactions. For a patient to say that he feels like his life is crumbling apart, that someone in his life is twisted, that things are chaotic, etc., is an invitation to create a visual image of this state or process.[12] This picture can sometimes be worked with through introjection into the body and sometimes through eliciting ego and object statements. For example, the crumbling metaphor can lead to something in which the image seems like a symbol (i.e. a generic wall that is crumbling) and another client may associate it with the crumbling ruins of Machu Picchu. With the latter, the patient's description of the place as beautiful, special, and their vocalized pity for its destruction by careless and greedy people can become relevant for an ego/object statement (i.e. Does it feel true for a part of you, if you say "I am beautiful, I am special, but you are careless and greedy, you are destroying me?"). Additionally, when a patient projects out a picture of her physical sensations, a fantasy or story can be created. Again, this is something that my patients started doing or hinted at themselves, and that I now introduce as an exercise with some who do not show the disposition to do so on their own. Lastly, as a principle, instead of fighting feelings or expressing them half way, it is much more efficacious to fully let them in. As opposed to asking a depressed patient to struggle and fight the fatigue, for example, fully allowing them to collapse and give in to the fatigue will allow another part of them to organically come out. I would like to share a clinical example that showcases a few of these things:

> Client comes in and reports that an ex-boyfriend is going to prison and focuses most of her attention on how his new girlfriend hates her. She strangely goes back and forth about how this girlfriend is jealous of her, but that she is skinny while client isn't and so she shouldn't be. I point out that attraction can be very different for some people. Client accepts this, but again wants to point out that she doesn't think she's traditionally beautiful. I agree that certain types of people might have classical beauty, but I ask client if she thinks she isn't attractive? Client says that she feels like she's attractive, but then adds that she thinks her personality makes her more so. I ask her to make her best guess about what the girlfriend might think about her.

She says, "you are intimidating in who and what you are, you want to steal my man, I'm jealous." I ask her to say these as ego and object statements, but change "steal my man" to "take what's mine." She tells me that a different ex-boyfriend and her sister come up. Because of recent work on this ex-boyfriend, I ask client to begin with him and she gives me a mock angry look, which is a game she often plays while doing this work with me. I meet her look with humor and her resistance goes away and she agrees to tell me what makes these statements feel true with him.

Client says she was "jealous of what he has and how he gets it," and recounts how he made a lot of money selling drugs, had people "convinced he was great," and people who "stood up for him." She tells me how he used to take her money from work, and the drugs that she got on her own, and hold on to them for her. She says that he would "feed them" to her at certain times and compares him to a "ruler, a dictator, who wants to control you and micro-manage everything you do." I ask her to focus on seeing him as this dictator and the associated memories and see which come most into focus. After BLS, she quickly reports that anger comes up and that she feels it in her chest and shoulders. I ask her to see how it wants to be expressed and she surprisingly says as "an explosion" that "happens inward." I ask her how it might look if it happened outwards and she looks, with seriousness, and says, "[she] could stab him." I explain to her that if she doesn't discharge this anger, that it is going to continue to explode in her and she agrees to picture him in their old place, in some prone position, and express it. However, after beginning BLS, she begins to move her mouth around and the serious determination begins to melt away. She eventually stops me and reports that she "do[es]n't ever see him anymore" and that she "can't picture him." She says that she "can feel him, but never tr[ies] to visualize him." I ask "can't or won't?" With some seriousness, she says that she doesn't want to picture him. I ask her to finish the sentence, "If I let myself visualize him, then I might . . . " She takes a minute and I see a smile come across her face quickly once or twice, and I ask her to "spit it out." She groans and says, with exasperation, "surrender, cave in." She quickly says that she's "mad" that with all the progress that she's made, that she would still feel this way. I clarify that it's only a part of her, but she says that he'll be getting out of prison soon and it frustrates her to think of crossing paths with him in the near future and how everything she's worked on could "go down the drain." I see frustration in her and ask her to picture him and see if that part of her that wants to surrender is really greater than the part that is angry at all he had done to her. She agrees to try, but before I begin BLS she tells me that she could tell that she'd lose her anger once she pictures him.

I ask client to associate to explosion and to tell me the first thing that comes to mind when she pictures an explosion. She has a slightly disgusted look and says that she pictures a body exploding and "splattering" everywhere. I ask her to picture it and see what gets more of her focus, the explosion itself or the splattering. She says the latter and says she pictures the skin in "little, itty bitty, bloody pieces." I ask her to picture them in her shoulders and chest and see if they feel right there. She again gives me a mock angry look and then follows the BLS. She quickly says it doesn't feel right, but I ask her to give it a better try. She has a look of surprise and says it feels right in the back of her shoulders. After they fully embed, she tells me that her body reacts and she feels like her back wants to arch. I ask her if she has a sense of how she could literally move into an arch position, but she tries to explain how she doesn't think it's possible. I don't really understand, but she seems to be honest here, and so I ask her to project it out. She tells me that she sees a hunched-back person. I ask her "man, woman, child . . . ?" and she responds with "old man." I ask her about his facial expression and she says that he is "miserable." I ask for clarification and she says "sad and angry." I ask her if she feels like the image wants to change or express an action and she says that it doesn't but doesn't seem sure.

I ask her to fast forward the image a few minutes, a few hours, and then a few days and see if she has a sense for any changing wanting to come out. She then says that she pictures him walking by himself and that he stays away from people and hides in the shadows. I ask her where she pictures him and she says "in a city" on "a gloomy day and no one's around." I ask her to imagine that someone comes into the scene and if it is a man, woman, child, animal . . . and she says a woman. I ask her what happens when she begins to get close to him. She says he backs up and disappears. I ask her what the woman's thoughts about this are. She says, that the woman saw him, tried to get to him, in order to "see that he's ok." I ask why she had concern, and client tells me that she saw that he looked upset. I ask if the sadness or anger was what she wanted to check on, and she says that the sadness is bigger in him.

I ask her to make statements about the hunchback from the place of the woman and she says, "you are hiding, you don't want to be found, I don't feel good, I feel sorry for him." I ask her to put these into ego and object statements about someone from her past, and she says that her mother and her biological father come to mind. I ask her to focus on both and see who she feels more strongly about, and she says her mother. She reports several memories and I ask her to focus on them and see which one is strongest. After I begin BLS, I see her mouth moving again and can tell she's blocking feelings. I ask her to focus on her mouth and the block and feel the tensions in her mouth and see if she can get a sense for how much of her face that it affects. She reports that it stays around her mouth and I ask her to project out the sensations. She says that she pictures a black hole. I ask her to see if it fits in or around her mouth. She says it does, and then I get her to embed it. Afterwards she can feel some anger arising towards her mother, but says that it is like she is wearing "a muzzle" and can't say anything to her. I ask her to picture the muzzle on her and she says it feels right. I ask her to see how her body reacts and she reports more anger coming up. I ask her what is stronger the anger, or the part that wants to surrender and be "an obedient dog." She looks at me with mock anger that lasts a little longer than usual. We continue BLS for a while but eventually she tells me that the anger dies down and she "can't say anything yet." She then says that she feels exhausted, and wants to just "spill onto the floor." Because I've seen this before, I ask her to let this part express itself and to picture herself becoming a puddle in her mind's eye. I begin BLS, tell her to let this mindset take her over and to see if it feels right to spill into a puddle. She says it feels right to become one, during the BLS, and after a minute or so she breaks BLS to express with surprise that it feels like she has "no words" to express the state that she's in. I tell her to just enjoy the comfort in not struggling to keep a shape, and to just wait and see if her body or mind starts to react to this state.

She makes another face that communicates she is frustrated. I tell her to just stick with the feelings and then to project them out. She says that she pictures a tall geyser. I ask her how tall and she tells me that it's bigger than trees in the forest and says "waterfall tall" as if this is a meaningful comparison. I ask her to see if she can picture it inside of her body and if there's a place it feels right. She tells me that it feels right in her stomach. She uncomfortably laughs as soon as I begin the BLS, and her eyes look at me with a strange intensity. She says that she pictures it erupting out of her mouth. I ask her to stay with it, and let it embed and soon she tells me that it feels like she wants to "puke." I ask her to stay with it and to tell me if the nausea grows. She tells me that it does after a few more passes of BLS, and I ask her to discharge it by imagining she is vomiting in her mind's eye. She agrees and after I resume BLS, I tell her that as she's "puking" that she should see if someone shows up on the other end, and to tell me who she wants to puke on. She says that it's her mother and client smiles and nervously laughs as she discharges it. When it's fully discharged she says that her puking felt like words. She reports that she is calm and that she felt pent up before and now it's gone. She says that she still feels like the geyser is in her, but that she doesn't feel any pressure or tension from it. She reports that she can feel the well-being in her stomach and we anchor it to a memory from her past.

Some readers may feel that this session was chaotic and the technique too unstructured (i.e. I am jumping from one thing to another). My only defense is that this patient, like many others, has a strong aggression block from early superego development, and she needed to discharge it. Without doing so such patients cannot process the material and themes that initially arose in the session. Imagining herself as a puddle and the id aggression of vomiting, allowed my patient to access very primitive superego relations. Accessing and processing conflict within these areas of development can have the most significant global effects on someone's character. Once this seal is broken, a patient is able to begin discharging and processing more aggression, in a more steady and linear way.[13] In creating a story around the projection, patients will often bring in other characters that provide an inter-relation from which to generate ego and object statements, leading to real events or relations from their past. These techniques have also been valuable in creating fantasies that lead to an anxiety situation to which the patient can react. Sometimes emotions or specific id drives will spontaneously arise in the fantasy, and they can be discharged there or, more classically, used in transference interpretations. Moreover, depressive patients who have become puddles, like the one from this example, have gone on to become pumpkins or a plant, while some have become cubes or some other form with depth. Many will also describe a "bounce back" to take a full human form again in the same session. There is often development in symbols and, on their own, some patients will find a way to incorporate them in their life outside of the clinic. As with much else, I sometimes take their habits or practices, and suggest them to some patients who I think would be open to such ideas.

Lastly, it is very important that this clinical approach is not treated as a gimmick. If one does not put work into the therapeutic alliance, patients will not be willing to enter the overwhelming feelings of the initial ego injuries. For some patients, it takes many sessions beyond the 12 or 20 sessions of short-term treatment to begin to use these techniques. Somatic approaches have concepts like grounding and work with the breath to strengthen a patient, and, for some patients, this approach cuts past a lot of the intellectualization or superficial content with which some begin treatment. However, some people must first be approached from the mind/personality and they are very uncomfortable focusing on their bodies or being looked at in this way. Additionally, even when staying verbal, there are some patients with whom one cannot ask many questions or, initially, disrupt their narrative. In short, there is no getting around long-term therapy in many cases, nor established training that allows a psychotherapist to properly conceptualize the building of the therapeutic alliance.[14]

Notes

1 There are also many variations of how one should use the transference. Some analysts hold that one leaves a positive transference going and work through the negative transference, instead of interpreting whatever transference comes up. Some analysts focus not on interpreting the transference being replayed but advocate that the analyst should play it in a new way. Some analysts focus on the curative properties of the transference and how, without real action, the analyst should play into the transference until the patient overcomes it himself. There are many schools of psychoanalysis and many more ways to look at and work with transference in the clinic.

2 In Chapters 5 and 6 this will be investigated more formally in the concepts of the proto, deutero, and trito relation to the parental imago.

3 In *The Economics of Libido* (2015) I bring up Abram Kardiner's criticism of Freud's idea that psychosexual development is static and universal in the conclusion. Kardiner (1939) invokes the absence of anal traits in several primitive political economies, and raises the question of how anality could be linked to satisfaction in certain intellectual abilities and behaviors. I suggest that it is important to recognize a Marxian approach in which the development of technology and class struggle play a role. For example, the technology for more complex housing is needed before a chief removes himself from the tribe that he rules, declares himself taboo, becomes guarded and removed from the people, and creates a structural position of power in discourse. This relation to authority, which illustrates

how a regular human being can receive a transference that makes him or her seem much more perfect, powerful, or magical, is not universal or part of every political economy. In the slavery and domination, which would go into creating it, we have a likely candidate for the linking of anality, for example, to certain pleasures—the pleasures that slaves would have to learn to enjoy in order to make the best of an intolerable situation.

4 There used to be a time in which analysts like Melanie Klein (1932, 1975) and Ives Hendrick (1936), for example, were trying to categorize psychopathology based upon id drives. Klein (1928), very early in her writings, linked id drive, parental imago, superego, and Oedipus complex: "analysis of little children reveals the structure of the super-ego as built up of identifications dating from very different periods and strata in the mental life. These identifications are surprisingly contradictory in character, over-indulgence and excessive severity existing side by side. We find in them, too, an explanation of the severity of the super-ego, which comes out specially plainly in these infant analyses. It does not seem clear why a child of, say, four years old should set up in his mind an unreal, phantastic image of parents who devour, cut and bite. But it *is* clear why in a child of about *one year* old the anxiety caused by the beginning of the Oedipus conflict takes the form of a dread of being devoured and destroyed. The child himself desires to destroy the libidinal object by biting, devouring and cutting it, which leads to anxiety, since awakening of the Oedipus tendencies is followed by introjection of the object, which then becomes one from which punishment is to be expected. The child then dreads a punishment corresponding to the offence: the super-ego becomes something which bites, devours and cuts" (p. 168).

5 This defense has also been described as moving from passive (victim) to active (perpetrator) but, as will be shown, the individual can also move from active to passive in this sense and what remains constant is the object playing the role of the self imago. I will take up Klein's use of PI more in Chapter 5.

6 The importance of perfection has always been around in clinical concepts like megalomania, narcissism, etc. but death hasn't received the same importance. The work of Eigen (1995, 2004) on aliveness and deadness, and Green (1997) on the dead mother were very suggestive when I was thinking through these issues. When I re-introduce psychic bisexuality in the next book, I will have more to say about the ties of the parental imago of death to the passive-altruistic pole of development, as well as the dialectical syntheses of the poles of perfection and death.

7 Once I more formally introduce the psychoanalytic model of mind in Chapters 5 and 6, I will take up this early relation and show how psychopathology shows up in both external and internal Space.

8 In the face of being "cut off," or no longer "enabled," by others who have made one feel entitled or accustomed to the help, many patients do not feel like they deserved it. Instead, these types of memories can often lead the person to holding resentment towards the parent or parental-substitute.

9 Sometimes fully embedding a symbol will lead to a memory from childhood to emerge, sometimes a part of the patient that wants to reject the image can be used to create a new memory network, and sometimes feeling spontaneously emerges.

10 "This result may be produced by anything that causes the libido to flow backwards (i.e. that causes a 'regression'): whether, on the one hand, the libido becomes collaterally reinforced owing to some disappointment over a woman, or is directly dammed up owing to a mishap in social relations with other men—both of these being instances of 'frustration'; or whether, on the other hand, there is a general intensification of the libido, so that it becomes too powerful to find an outlet along the channels which are already open to it, and consequently bursts through its banks at the weakest spot" (Freud, 1911b, p. 62).

11 The shared imagos from childhood development and the mimetic sense are what allow for symbols to be created that have trans-historical meaning across cultures. This is usually taken as the domain of Jung, but Freud (1911b) is not opposed to it: "Since I published my work upon Schreber, a chance acquisition of knowledge has put me in a position to

appreciate one of his delusional beliefs more adequately, and to recognize the wealth of its bearing upon *mythology* ... [M]y analysis of a paranoid patient may serve to show that Jung had excellent grounds for his assertion that the mythopoeic forces of mankind are not extinct, but that to this very day they give rise in the neuroses to the same psychical products as in the remotest past ages" (pp. 80–82).

12 Freud (1900) shows that words can become pictures in a rebus, and a conversion symptom in the body can be related to words. In full parallelism, words can become symbols, and the repression of id impulses in the physical suppression that shows up in the chronic muscular tension, for example, how a bodily zone can be related to symbols.

13 There is also the reverse, when a serious and cold patient is able to begin taking in aspects and feelings that are often cute, dopey, cuddly, and joyful.

14 I have to admit that I am saying this as an inexperienced clinician. Moreover, I should point out that I have met very talented therapists who can go very far in their verbal or somatic approaches. Still, I would venture that for the inexperienced and average psychotherapist, like myself, having the ability to use either a psychic or somatic approach allows for the therapeutic alliance to form sooner. Given the great differences between patients, providing training for both approaches seems like the most ethical and equitable stance for established programs.

2

THE MANIFEST DOUBLE AND THE UNCANNY

The symptom reading is a logical progression from the scholarly tradition of the literary double. Analysis of the double, from a modern, psychological view, begins with Otto Rank, and I will show the major touchstones from Rank onward. In this review, I will divide the analysis of the literature into three schools of scholarship. The first school deals with the manifest double: a supernatural manifestation of the duplication of the protagonist's body in an external character or several internal characters trying to control the protagonist's body. The second school deals with the latent double: a mode of interpretation wherein the protagonist is in a double relation with another character who need not physically resemble him or herself. Textual hints of shared identity, moral complementarity of good and evil, separated plots that allow for a juxtaposition, and other procedures are used in order to show how a protagonist, or another character in a text, may be doubled. The third school deals with the double as an avatar. This reading has been adopted by feminist criticism to argue that the oppressed consciousness of female characters has been displaced onto another character.

The manifest double

The analysis of the double begins with the fantastical creation of a character who is a physical duplicate of the protagonist (a doppelgänger), or a character that is divided into fully separate personalities (a dissociated identity). Dostoevsky's *The Double* (1846) and more subtly, the portrait in Oscar Wilde's *The Picture of Dorian Gray* (1890) portray an important and deadly relationship between the protagonist and another person or representation that looks just like him. Stevenson's *Strange Case of Dr. Jekyll and Mr. Hyde* (1886) is a popular, if not the idiomatic, example of this overt division of the mind. Instead of an external person who is one's physical duplicate, who the protagonist can see and with whom he or she can interact, one's mind is duplicated or another's mind enters one's body. However, the control that the other mind has over one's body, behaviors, or actions usually is not directly known. Variations exist, but these texts exemplify the basic formula.

Rank's pioneering work in *The Double* (1971) begins with the film, *The Student of Prague* (1913), and his study ranges through both high and popular cultural sources. Rank returns to his subject frequently, looking at the phenomenon widely in different mediums and historical forms in his search for the double's pre-modern antecedents. Since my concern is with the ideas and procedures of analysis, and not the scholarship of Rank himself, I will use whichever text has the strongest formulation of his interpretation of the double.

Rank's psychoanalytic analysis of the double takes several forms. The first is psychobiography of the author. He notes that some of the authors whose work he looks at display "psychic disturbances or neurological and mental illnesses, and during their lifetime they demonstrated a marked eccentricity in behavior" (Rank, 1971, p. 35). While it is legitimate to say that an author's creations should reflect his own psychology, it is outside the scope of this project to argue that the screenwriter or the director involved in a film has shown eccentric behavior, gone to a therapist, or is on medication for a diagnosed mental health issue. The second foundation comes from Rank's link of the modern literary double to folk tales, superstitions, and myths of the past. Rank holds that some beliefs found in early cultures, such as not letting one's shadow fall upon a dead person, coffin, or tomb for fear that it will infect one with death, or fear of magic being used against one's shadow, reveal elements consistent with a double. The shadow is treated as a physical embodiment of the individual's soul and this mirrors how the death of the double in nineteenth-century stories lead to the death of the protagonist. There are many interesting examples and variations of this that he provides. For example, in certain cultures photography was linked to magical control of the soul of the person who is photographed. Rank provides ethnographical evidence that some cultures formally separate the shadow soul from another soul in the individual. One soul was tied up with the idea of immortality and life after death, but the other soul was part of an individual's experiences with magic, or in later developments, it is connected with "the world of dreams" and aspects of both the cognitive and emotional life of the individual (Rank, 1941, p. 75).

Rank's textual analysis of the double creates the opposition of *the social self* to impulses that would transgress laws or mores in one's culture and community. In *The Student of Prague* (1913), Rank gives us the example of a student who sells his mirror reflection to the devil, who becomes his double and interferes with his social ambitions and amorous affairs. Eventually, the double frustrates him enough that he is effectively driven to suicide by killing the double. Rank (1941) holds that the moral is that "a man's past—represented in the film by the hero's own youthful image—is so intimately bound to his vital being that misfortune befalls him if he tries to detach himself too completely from it" (p. 69). I understand this as the idea that when an individual does not have his or her worth confirmed by significant figures, that ambitions or getting self-esteem from sexual conquests, for example, can become valorized. One was treated unfairly or wrongly attacked, but one is not worthless if one is rich, has a prestigious job, has unlocked the secrets of the Bible, or is desired by the opposite sex. This valorization to save self-worth is comparable to "a deal with the devil" in that these pursuits for gaining self-esteem are themselves subject to ego injuries (social humiliations, disappointments in love, etc.). To encounter such injuries means that these strategies will be repressed and have defenses enacted against them, which invites "the devil" of mental illness into one's life.

For Rank (1941), the double is not only the youthful image of the individual that emerges in his "personal past" but is an evil, criminal, or even "silly" or "funny" self that is "repudiated by the social self" (p. 82). He notes megalomanic paranoia in some versions, forms in which the double is a "guardian angel," as well as some in which the protagonist's identity become confused with the double (ibid., p. 70). Despite recognizing these variations due to individual psychology, Rank stresses that the stereotypical modern double has received a moralistic interpretation and is the harbinger of the individual's death in many novels. In contrast, the double of primitive political economies was viewed as a protecting force. Rank links this change to the advent of Christianity and its doctrine of heaven and hell, which illustrates preoccupation with sin and bad conscience. This view of the individual can be contrasted to former conceptions of the afterlife. For example, the underworld governed by Hades in Greek mythology was not a place of torture or punishment for the guilty dead, but was instead where the majority of the undistinguished dead would go in contrast to the Elysian fields or Tartarus.

Rank's idea of relating the nineteenth-century double to the Christian worldview roughly follows Freud's idea of worldviews in history illustrating how the superego develops in children. Freud (1913) famously divides worldviews into a stage of animism, then religion, and a final stage of science (p. 88). He regards this cultural progression as an illustration of the increasing object relatedness of the child. It first relates to impersonal forces and impersonal things in its environment, with the parental caregivers being taken for granted (i.e. a baby dies without the administrations of its parents). Increasing cognitive capacities that follow the object relations of the child, allow it to begin to form a more human and nuanced view of itself and others. The child's egocentrism, and the idealization of itself or its caregivers are eventually overcome as illustrated in the requirements of reproducibility in science. Testing a hypothesis in a way that others can repeat, illustrates both humility and a sense of protection in the pursuit of knowledge. It is humble to put forward knowledge that must be validated by others, and challenging the knowledge claim of others through this framework helps to work against tendencies to idolize an intellectual figure or fear their disapproval.

The Christianity of the nineteenth century illustrates very strong object relatedness in its injunctions to love one's neighbor and in its prohibitions against sinning against them. However, in contrast to science, Christianity and other religions still invoke the perfection, infallibility, and incontestability of deities and their earthly representatives. In contrast to these religions, the fetish objects, animals, and environmental forces in animism are emphasized, with less "humanistic" injunctions to relate to others and less subtle prohibitions of what constitutes sinning against others. Additionally, the catastrophes of events like eclipses and droughts, which are tied to moral transgressions in animism, gradually disappear in religions and the power of humans in this world is reduced. This does not mean that there are not animistic qualities in monotheistic religions, for example, or humanistic qualities in animistic religions. As with the issues of the confluence of many drives, ideals, and fantasies over-determining an action or symptom in psychoanalysis, it is a matter of recognizing the emphasis of certain material. A linear developmental pattern is present in this emphasis, but both progressive and regressive trends appear to blur its outline. More will be said about object relations when I formally look at Freud's examination of the double and the uncanny.

Rank (1971) applies psychoanalytic theory to the manifest double in three main ways. First, the social self inhibits certain desires that become projected into the double. There are some important clarifications between shame, guilt, and inner vs. outer inhibitions on one's desires that Rank does not analyze. I will attempt to introduce them in latter chapters, but, regardless, Rank holds that the double is the personification of the desires that were felt to be unacceptable and that are now satisfied in it, "without responsibility" (ibid., p. 76). Second, Rank holds that "a powerful fear of death" is involved in the creation of the double, which he links to the fear of "the expectation of the unavoidable destiny of death" (ibid., p. 77). Rank argues against the instinct of self-preservation as underlying this fear of death, and instead quotes a psychologist who finds a "love for the personality peculiar to [the individual], found in his conscious possession . . . the central self of his individuality, which attaches him to life" (ibid., p. 78). Rank matches this to the stage of narcissism in psychosexual development, but he expands on this stage to also include things like the idealism/solipsism of certain types of philosophers who believe that the external world may be something that just exists in their own minds. It is improbable that this perception or fantasy of the philosopher is one that everyone has, and since Rank points to a special self-love that is not part of the regular self-preservation anxiety, there is likely a non-universal phase in play. Rank does not make this conceptual distinction in his work, but I will attempt to do so in the latter chapters of this book. Third, Rank interprets that there is both defensive self-love in the protagonist and that his self-hate is put into the double. "An erotic attitude toward one's own self," he writes, "is only possible because along with it the defensive feelings can be discharged by way of the hated and feared double" (ibid.). In this formulation, Rank is very close to spelling out the defense of projective identification, which I covered in the previous chapter. However, since he does not formally investigate other examples of the double (ex. the guardian angel), or show a similar structure of projective identification in them, I question how conscious he is of a formal mechanism.

Lastly, Rank (1971) expands manifest doubling past a shared body, or duplication of one's body, in his analysis of Dostoevsky's *The Brothers Karamazov* (1880). Since fantastical duplicates represent the base or bad impulses that are repressed in the protagonist, Rank (1971) argues that shared blood or familial bonds also allow a brother, twin sister, etc. to serve a similar function (p. 75). An early critic who comments on Rank, Ralph Tymms (1949), builds on Rank's view here by spelling out the connection of Smerdyakov to Ivan. The latter corrupts the former with his "blasphemous arguments," and Tymms argues for a "spiritual affinity" between the two by noting Ivan's many thoughts of, and reactions to Smerdyakov (ibid., pp. 100–101). I will turn to the work of Tymms in a moment, but I include him here because I want to make sure that I provide textual examples of how critics propose we understand doubling. Ultimately, the invocation of a shared body (one body with several minds or one that is duplicated) along with the extension of the physical body through familial/blood ties, is the structure of the first school of double scholarship.

Tymms (1949) expands on Rank's presentation in some interesting ways. He includes some stories of mesmerism in which one person has the power to control the mind of another and be that person's second self. Additionally, along with the examples of one's mirror reflection and shadow representing one's "soul self" in early cultures, Tymms brings up the werewolf or wizard taking animal form. "The truant spirit," he writes "masquerading as a wer-animal, involves its owner in the injuries which may result from its adventures" (ibid., p. 18). Tymms goes on to enumerate myths or fables of animals being changed into men to serve as doubles of humans, and stories of wizards or goblins who impersonate men. Additionally, gods and supernatural deities can also take mortal form and be guardian angels or doubles, triples, quadruples, etc. of mortals for their own amorous interest in an earthly woman (ibid., p. 20). Tymm's brings up instances of the magical renewal of youth and other magical effects that could count as variations of the double theme, but it is outside the scope of this review to give an exhaustive catalogue of his findings.

Along with showing that Rank's focus on the fantastical is too narrow, Tymms also criticizes him for basing his interpretation of the double on the theme of narcissism, or "elements of morbid self-love." This latter criticism seems uncharitable since Rank is focused on the "modern" double and he does not claim that the shadow or mirror image of earlier times was related to morbid self-love. Additionally, Rank does not claim that the double he focused on in the nineteenth and twentieth century was the only type. As mentioned above, he notes a "guardian angel" version, although he doesn't formally investigate it. In Rank's last words on the subject, in *Beyond Psychology* (1941), he stresses poles of "likeness and difference" in the personality (pp. 99–100), which seem comparable to the poles of activity and passivity that I will examine in the next book. Such a division would put morbid self-love in the pole of difference and allow for other manifestations in the pole of likeness. Tymms' focus on other types outside the trend of the time is welcome, but his criticism of Rank appears to be a strawman for the psychoanalytic interpretation. Although, one cannot be too critical of the caricatures of psychoanalysis when they are partly invited by the use of vague and undefined concepts.

Rosemary Jackson's (1986) "Narcissism and Beyond" follows Rank and Tymms in looking at the fantastic double. In this case, it follows their formula of familial ties allowing for a double in the novel of *Frankenstein* (1822). Her study is of note because it is an early attempt to bring a Lacanian lens to the subject. Jackson follows Rank as seeing desire that opposes the inhibition of the social self, or social convention, leading to a deflection of desire into the "weird, refracted world" of the fantastic double. She contrasts earlier versions of the double as allegories of good and evil with the idea that more psychological versions of the doppelgänger illustrate "a quest for wholeness and integration" (Jackson, 1986, p. 45). She acknowledges object relations in Freud's classic model, and sketches a rough model of a narcissistic stage of self-love or primary narcissism, a stage of attachment to objects, and a third stage of "the acceptance of the laws of the world" that tie to "self-repression for the sake of cultural continuity" (ibid., p. 46). Between the first and second stages she inserts Lacan's mirror stage as the alienation in which the self is recognized as separate from the object through "the look" or gaze of the object. The former sense of the body, before the mirror stage, consists of a body of "fragments" which she relates to Frankenstein's monster: sewn together from different corpses and initially having no language. She holds that there is a desire to leave the awareness of the self as separate, which was an awareness constituted through the gaze of the other to make an ideal ego, and that this desire can have a regressive pull on the self.

Jackson holds that Lacan treats this desire to leave awareness of the self as the "central unconscious longing in every human being" and compares it to the mystical desire for oneness with God (ibid., p. 46). The mirror image becomes the visual representation of the feeling that one's essence, which is held in the body, cannot be truly enclosed within this limited space. She combines this with Rank's idea of the double as constituting immortality and thus a denial of the power of death. In her example of *Frankenstein*, the doctor's obsession with the monster he created is an internal one and Jackson indicates that the doctor's death and the monster's vanishing into the ice and snow illustrates the "radical open-endedness of being" (ibid., p. 49). This dissatisfaction with embodiment itself is an antecedent of dissatisfaction with cultural laws. Although she initially billed the double as a quest for wholeness and integration, Jackson quotes Irving Massey near the end of her article to express how both Frankenstein and his monster will "resume their endless dialectic of conflict, until, in death, they spiral into one again" (p. 50). The wholeness can never be attained and the inner excess in the human being will always push beyond any established boundary.

Although Jackson's article is an enjoyable glance at the double, there are good reasons to doubt the originality of the Lacanian contribution to the psychoanalytic theory. Rank, Freud, and other early analysts have already noted dynamics with the mirror image, longing for immortality, anxieties of bodily instability, or primary narcissistic states like "oceanic oneness," which make a Lacanian claim to originality here very dubitable. Lacan's early claim of the mirror's literal role in early development is an original contribution, but, as Norman Holland (1998) points out, the childhood observation literature doesn't support Lacan's claim about the child of 6–18 months finding "jubilation" in its own image. The child's consciousness of its own mirror image only arises in the second half of this period (i.e. 12–18 months) and according to Holland's citation of Mahler and others, the children "do not show the jubilation Lacan claims" (ibid., sec. III). Moreover, Lacan (1998) himself brings up the criticism of how a blind infant will progress through the psychosexual stages without being able to see his or her mirror image, and drops the literal reference to the mirror image in his later work (pp. 92–93). This is a retraction of his specific contribution to the development of narcissism and really makes the point moot. Below, I will argue that projective identification with the parental imago constitutes the link that Rank finds between an individual and his shadow, picture image, mirror image, or double.

There is a problem for Lacanian interpretations that valorize anti-humanism and the desire to leave awareness of the self. I would like to preface this criticism by acknowledging that academic interpretations of Lacan do not necessarily follow how Lacanian clinicians interpret him. Regardless, Lacanian interpretations often do not show an understanding of the operations of defense. When therapists are able to undo such a defense, by working through the anxiety that caused it, the dialectic of Frankenstein and his monster comes to an end. This is not to say that the individual becomes "whole" in some metaphysical sense, but just that symptoms can be resolved: both ego alien ones and the "character armor" of projective identifications. Moreover, just as the projective identification that underlies the double can be resolved, as I will show below, there is more subtle pathology that Lacanian accounts like Jackson's do not identify in their valorization of excess. For example, triangular repetitions with parental-substitutes aren't visible in every individual: not every grad student is defiant or submissive with their professors, for example. For those who do exhibit these repetitions, this behavior was not always there with teachers/authorities in their past. Thus, there is a state of eros or fusion with parental imagos that can become defused so that triangular patterns emerge. A goal of analysis is to help the patient overcome such patterns, which are often tied to self-sabotaging impulses and seldom help them achieve the goals that they espouse.

In the Lacanian critique of ego psychology, the latter is often caricatured as conformity with societal norms, and submission to current power/authority structures. However, there is no virtue in rebellion or defiance that uncritically dismisses authority. For example, the high school dropout who feels that there is nothing important to learn in school and that he is smarter than everyone else, is no hero. Although he may have a sense of the "radical open-endedness of his being," how much of that experience is produced with drugs, and accompanied by destructiveness and mental pathology? The valorization of excess and radical open-endedness strikes me as a much more romantic notion than the humanism that came before. Although, just like the swing from Victorian sexual repression, to the sexual revolution of the 1960s and current casual attitudes about sex, there are obvious dialectical structures at work in society. The swing from humanism to anti-humanism is one such movement that begs for a synthesis.

Freud (1919b) offers both a summary and clarification of Rank's findings. Like Rank, he agrees that the shadow, mirror, and soul images of early cultures are an expression of primary narcissism reacting to fears of death, resulting in intimations of immortality. However, Freud more formally links autoscopy, or the perception of something that looks like oneself, to an aspect of the superego. It is comparable to other mental pathologies, like depersonalization or delusions of observation, from which Freud (1914a, 1919b, 1921) originally hypothesized the "over-I" and formalized "self-consciousness" as a separate psychic agency in the ego. Although autoscopy comes from an early stage of development, Rank's perception of the destiny of death cannot. Anxiety related to non-being, annihilation, etc. can be felt subjectively, but there cannot be anything resembling objective knowledge of death until more object relatedness enters development. Physical destructiveness, such as wanting to cannibalize someone or wishing that he or she would disappear are one thing, but the death of another implies a more nuanced reality principle in which the irreversibility of death and the recognition of the individuality of the other is appreciated.[1] The modern double, who represents the doom of its originator, must reference a confluence of superego reactions from both higher and lower stages. Freud's next point is also quite interesting:

> But it is not only this latter material, offensive as it is to the criticism of the ego which may be incorporated in the idea of a double. There are also all the unfulfilled but possible futures to which we still like to cling in [f]antasy, all the strivings of the ego which adverse external circumstances have crushed, and all our suppressed acts of volition which nourish in us the illusion of Free Will.
>
> *(Freud, 1919b, p. 236)*

Along with the vertical axis of superego development throughout childhood, Freud invokes a horizontal axis of different ego and object drives that can also be expressed through the double. This is the idea that people do not choose to be ambitious, compassionate, gregarious, controlling, etc., but are *driven* to be so, which makes free will an illusion. These various social drives are part of an individual's "psychical constitution [which] will play a decisive part, irrespectively of the external circumstances" (Freud, 1930, pp. 83–84). Of course, a given historical culture may, through the discipline and punishment of parents and authorities, mold its children towards certain ideals, and produce a second nature. However, this process can hardly explain the many differences that exist between individuals within a culture, or within a single family in which the children received the same instruction and discipline. As noted, Rank himself brings up the poles of likeness and difference in the personality, and these, along with Freud's poles of activity/passivity, are attempts to make sense of different types of motivational structures in individuals. I hope to make some conceptual clarifications in this important area in the next book.

Freud (1911b) initially introduces narcissism as a stage in which the child takes its own body as an object. This is illustrated in sexual perversions in which someone might masturbate to his own image in a mirror, or more mildly in watching himself in a mirror during sex with another. Freud (1914a) also extends it in the idea of narcissistic object-choice in which sexual desire and/or love seeks someone that reminds one of "(a) what he himself is (i.e. himself), (b) what he himself was" (Freud, 1914a, p. 90).[2] Freud (1914a) contrasts this to anaclitic object-choice, which is based on sexual or loving feelings being based on the prototype of one's caregivers. The first form of narcissistic object-choice is classically related to one of the earliest forms of homosexual desire. Freud (1922) articulates it in how a man "identifies himself with his mother, and looks about for love-objects in whom he can re-discover himself, and whom he might then love as his mother loved him" (p. 230). This can be understood as being in PI with a parental imago and for object-choice to be routed through this, towards the self imago. This form of narcissistic object-choice isn't exclusively homosexual and I have worked with both hetero and homosexual patients who have exhibited it. What is at stake is that a person is attracted to someone who literally looks like them (same eyes, same high cheekbones, etc.), shares their interests/likes, and has similar socioeconomic status (i.e. education, or income, etc.).[3] I have worked with many patients who have used the term "soul mate" to essentially describe this. They show up to a session and explain to me that another addict, who they just met, likes the same music they do, has the same sense of humor as they do, grew up in the same type of broken home, etc. Often this isn't the first time that they have found a soul mate, and this pattern can be explored through many relationships.

The second form of Freud's narcissistic object-choice shows up clinically as the projective identification of either the active or passive pole, or part of one's personality associated with too much bad conscience. I have had many female patients begin treatment by telling me that they want to leave the man who is either cheating on them, using them, threatening them, or giving them emotional or physical abuse. With such patients, I had previously tried to analyze their different motivations or fears. This was done with the thought that maybe they didn't think they could do better than this man, that they might have had their self-esteem ruined, or that they were altruistically sacrificing themselves for him. Even after a session that seemed to go well, a patient might have expressed the idea that she would leave him, kick him out, or separate, but invariably she did not, or she allowed him to come back later if she did.

There are many different defenses that are in play in abusive relationships, but two techniques highlight the second version of narcissistic object-choice involved in some of them. In the first, the same adjectives that she can use to describe her romantic partner, will apply to her in the past. For example, several female patients have focused on how breaking up with their boyfriend would mean that he would be homeless. Seeing the emphasis on this outcome, one can ask them if it feels true for a part of them to say, "I deserve to be homeless?" When one has built up enough rapport with them, and they have been able to adequately express how stuck they feel, then this can often trigger important material to come out. Material about being mean to an ex or using her parents will often come up. Other patients in similar relationships will describe how calling the police on their boyfriend is useless because "he's ruthless, above the law, he can manipulate them and anybody else, and always gets what he wants." Again, when enough of a therapeutic alliance is built up, these patients are often able to say these as ego statements and get into how cruel and selfish they had been with others in the past.[4] Here is a clinical example:

> Client tells me how she's decided not to make her boyfriend go to counseling or do any of the things that the therapy group had recommended to her. He had cheated on client several times in the past, and more generally left her with most of the responsibilities at the house. When they had broken up before, he had even stayed in the house and made client and the kids find somewhere to live. I ask client why she has decided against the group's advice. She tells me that he knows that she will leave if he cheats on her again. I'm skeptical and ask her to imagine that she catches him with another woman and to tell him it's over, and to see if there's any part of her that resists cutting ties. After BLS, client says that she told him, but that a part of her felt that "separation feels like failure." I ask her to focus on this feeling and see where it shows up in her body. She tells me that she feels it in her chest. I ask her to see if it wants to grow or change at all and resume BLS. She tells me no and I ask her to project it out. She tells me that she pictures someone who just lost a race and is on her knees. She gestures, with her arms raised, and tells me that the person "looks like failure." I ask her to introject this image and she says it feels right to picture it in her chest. I tell her to let her sensations fully map on to the image and to tell me when it is fully embedded. Client signals to me that it's fully in and I ask her to tell me if her body or mind has any reaction to it. Client tells me that her body wants to reject it. I ask her to focus on this and she tells me that she feels it in her stomach and the sensation is beginning to rise up from there.
>
> I ask client to stay with the feeling of failure and to tell me when she's had it before. She tells me when her marriage failed. She quickly adds "he wouldn't grow up" in regards to her husband. She adds a few other memories that involved her parents during her teen years and one earlier than this. One of them was when she moved out when she was 15 and she left her brother with her mother. I ask her to start with the most recent memory. She tells me about how the relationship with her husband fell apart after a year of marriage and that he began telling her that he was exhausted after work and he didn't help with the children. She adds that she felt like she was taking care of him, as much as the baby. She goes on to report that he'd only last at jobs for a few weeks and then would find an excuse to quit. Things got so bad, she reports, that they lost their house, car, and were "living homelessly." She tells me that she's a "very proud person" and couldn't ask family or friends for help during this time. I ask her how much longer they stayed together and she tells me for another year. She tells me that the last straw is when he used his money to buy a truck instead of paying the electricity bill.

She tells me that she moved back in with her parents and "it really sucked." She says that after this he played "guilt games" with her so that he could see the kids more, even though he didn't pay any child support. She reports that that he would work under the table so that he wouldn't have to pay any money, complaining that DFS took too much of his paycheck. She tells me that things got to their worst when a family member was sick and she had to leave the kids with him so that she could visit her in the hospital. She says that her ex-husband asked her for money so that he and the kids could go out for lunch and then called half an hour after to say that she should come back because he didn't know what to do with the kids. She tells me that it was "fucking ridiculous" and that she feels anger coming up. I resume BLS and she tells me that she feels it in her stomach. I ask her to see how it wants to come out and she tells me that she wants to punch. I ask her to picture him in her mind's eye and to express her anger to him in words and then to express it physically if her body still wants it. After BLS she tells me that she yelled at him and then hit him and that he looked "pathetic." I ask her to picture him looking this way and to tell me what her reaction is. After BLS she tells me that she feels "disgust." I ask her to elaborate and she tells me that it's because "he's ok with his lifestyle, he's ok with the kids seeing him this way, and he will just give them things to make them want to be with him." She describes some of the gifts he's given and how they are probably "stolen" and that she fears that they'll want to live with him when they are older.

I ask her to say these thing as ego and object statements about her relation to her brother when she left: "I am pathetic, I'm ok with my lifestyle, I'm ok with my brother seeing me this way." She says it feels true and tells me about how she left her brother with her mother and "didn't protect him." She says that she had wanted a childhood but knew their mother wouldn't really be there for him, and that he'd have to "step up" without her. I resume BLS and she says that she feels shame, that "it's strong," and that what she did was "really wrong." She expresses how she had been taking care of everyone but got "resentful," "stopped caring," and then she "got to be a kid" and "make bad decisions." She briefly describes her drinking, sexual promiscuity, and drug use. I explain to her that if she knows that she wouldn't do this again if she could go back in time, that she can apologize, and if she believes herself, that her brother will forgive her. Client agrees to picture him in her mind's eye and articulate her apology. After BLS, she tells me that he accepted the apology but "he looks angry." I ask her to focus on his anger and see if she has a reaction to it. After BLS, she tells me that she feels guilt in her stomach and it's getting tighter. I resume BLS and tell her to stay with it until it's fully developed. After she signals me to stop, I ask her to project it out. She tells me that she sees a rope with many knots in it. I ask her to picture it in her stomach and to tell me if it feels right. During BLS she tells me that it feels right and I tell her to let me know when it's fully embedded. After it is in, I ask her if her body or mind has any reaction to it. She tells me that she "sense[s] that [she] deserves his anger." I ask her to say something more in her apology, something she didn't say last time, and see if this will work. After BLS, she tells me that he's now more understanding but "still angry though."

She begins to talk about how she felt a "sense of relief" in "not taking care of anyone" when she chose to "be a kid." She tells me that "everyone leaned on [her]" and that it "would get heavy." I ask her to focus on her brother's anger and to try to articulate what he was thinking about her. She comes up with, "you are selfish, I had to pick up that weight [that you left], you babied me, you kept me unaware of the full extent of the problems in our household . . . you protected me from the problem but then you just left." She finishes this off with, "I don't understand why." I ask client to say these as ego and object statements, about someone from her past. She tells me that her father comes to mind. She elaborates that he "kept [her] blind" and that when she found out that her siblings were being hurt and she was being protected by him that "it didn't make [her] feel happy . . . it made [her] feel worse." I resume BLS and she reports that she feels it in her chest and stomach and she feels "angry, worried, and disappointed." I ask her to express these feelings to the image of her father from this time and to see if he accepts it. After BLS, she tells me that "he didn't take it" and gets into how "everyone has to just go along with pretending that things happened the way he says they happened." I ask her if she has any insight into why he can't hear the truth? She tells me that "he doesn't want to feel the guilt."

I ask her to complete the sentence, "If I made him accept things as they really happened then he might . . ." She says "break." I do another: "If my father broke in accepting his guilt, then I might . . ." She says "feel bad." I ask her to focus on the part of her that wants him to admit the truth and the part that feels bad that he might break and see which feels stronger. After BLS she says that her "knowing is enough" and that "if he wants to pretend" she's ok with it. She adds that she "can't count [her]self higher than him" and "break him." I ask her if she can talk to him as an equal and let him know that both of them have to grow and to see whether they can help each other. She agrees to try this and I resume BLS. After, she tells me that he accepted it, but that it felt like he was "placating" her. She adds that "he's a good manipulator." I point out that she again can see through him and I tell her that if she doesn't stand up to him that she will never feel like her truth has a space to exist. I say that she doesn't have to ask him to admit he's wrong in front of anyone in real life, but that she deserves to have her own space where he can validate what she knows inside of her. Client agrees to try again and I resume BLS. After, she tells me that he "got angry" I ask her to picture this and see her reaction. After BLS, she tells me that she "just let go." She reports that she said, "this is what you did, what I know happened" and that he "looked scared . . . like he has no power." I ask her to look at his scared face and to see her reaction. After BLS, she says "part of

> [her] wants to go back" and "feels bad for hurting him." She says another part "feels strong . . . guilty, but strong." I ask her to stay with these two different parts of her and to not make a decision about what she will do, but to be prepared to talk about it more next session. She begins to cry and tells me that she knows that she's "not going to give in or go back [to him]." I pass her a tissue and wait silently until she's more composed and I tell her that I will see her next week.

My patient projected her bad, "kid" self, who abandoned her brother and chose to just live for her own fun, into boyfriends and husbands who treated her and their family with similar selfishness and indifference. This issue itself arose in PI and it had to be traced back further to when my patient felt the way her brother felt towards her, with their father. Additionally, just as she allowed her father's version of the past to reign, she often let her romantic partners gaslight her (i.e. make her question if her version of their misdeeds was accurate).

The other technique involves work through active imagination and corresponds to certain recurring symbols/bodily zones. The projection of the spine that goes along with strong inhibition of anger and assertiveness in the individual is very common, while the symbol of many "grabby" hands seems to be ubiquitous. For example, one female patient with a powerful aggression block, found it hard to even share her concerns that her partner was living off of her and wanted to dip into her savings.

> In the session in question, she gets to the point that she is able to express some anger towards him and calls her partner a "worthless jackass," but then quickly gets angry with herself for "being conned by him" and "taken down by him." She adds that she still had to make sure that she doesn't "fall for his traps," and take him back, otherwise he will continue to "be a burden on [her]." I ask her for an association to trap and she says an animal trap. I ask her for the first type of animal that came to mind and she says a lion. Then, she strangely adds that she can't let her partner continue to "eat her up." I ask her to imagine that she is trapped in a lion's mouth and begin BLS and ask her if any physical sensations or new thoughts come up. She says that she feels tension in her neck and shoulders. I have her exaggerate the tension by holding her shoulders up. She holds them up for half a minute and then reports feeling aggressive feelings "to punch" rise up in her.
>
> I put her back in the fantasy and ask her to begin in the lion's mouth but to see if she can get out and punch him on the nose to express the impulses. After BLS, she reports that she escaped and had clawed at the lion instead of punching it. She then reports that her partner appeared in the fantasy and began laughing at her. She says that it felt like her "power had left" and she felt "little" while he seemed "big" and "ferocious." I ask her to think of a powerful animal and she tells me that a bear comes to her mind. I ask her to imagine that she has a bear with her and to put herself back in the fantasy

with her "ferocious" partner and see if the bear makes her feel safe. I then ask her if she feels like she'd be able to unleash it on her partner if he continues to menace her.[5] I begin BLS and we resume the fantasy. After I stop the stimulation, she reports that she unleashed the bear on her partner but reports that it would "swipe" at her partner but then her partner would swipe at it, and they chased each other around without any resolution. I observe that it sounds like he's too powerful for any human or animal and she agrees with this. I ask her if she knows of anything that feels strong enough to take him on and she sullenly shakes her head no. I ask if he seems like a demon or maybe the devil, himself and she nods her head in the affirmative. In previous sessions, she mentioned the importance of her faith, so I ask her if she believes that God is powerful enough to deal with him and she says that He is. I ask her to imagine if something like a ray of light could come from the heavens to take care of the demon and I then begin BLS. After stopping me, she reports that a ray of light came from the clouds and split the earth and the demon/her partner fell inside of it, but only "partially." I ask why only "partially," and she says because a part of her didn't want to let him go and that she had imagined herself kicking at the earth and wants to kick him still. This develops into the idea that she wants to "win" and doesn't want to let him go because she wants to be the one to laugh last. We begin a discussion that leads back to her first husband and how he had hurt her and how she might not truly love her current partner. This seems like an important insight and discussion, but in previous experiences analysis of these things didn't change the ability of other patients to keep the man out of their lives, so I jot this down in my notes as something to return to later.

I ask client to return to the idea that her partner might be a demon, and for her to imagine what a demon looks like in its true form, when it isn't taking a human form like her boyfriend's body.[6] She says that the demon that comes to mind looks like an "alien" with "many, grabby arms." I ask her to picture the alien and its grabby hands and arms inside of her and to see if she could feel how her body wants to become like its body or make similar movements. I begin BLS and she begins to report during it that she feels the connection in her lower back. She then adds that she feels like her spine is getting bigger. When she stops the BLS, she reports that the alien image, and its power, had gone in all the way to her spine and that she feels "big." She then adds that she had imagined that her partner saw her grow and that he turned into "a puddle" in front of her, due to her sheer power. She then exclaims, "I hate him, everything he's done to me," and she says it with real conviction, which I have never seen in her before.

Like the first technique above, the insight into the defense is not enough. The overwhelming feelings and id drives that cause a patient to implement this defense, have to be processed. Otherwise, she can simply enact it again and project her bad conscience or her active/power pole into the love object. In the last clinical example of Chapter 1, instead of a giant demon or alien, a really "tall" geyser is what imparted the sense of height and power for that patient. This element, which ranges across several different forms, is likely the common denominator for the extreme aggression block. However, this puddle–great height dynamic has shown up without a severely codependent relationship being present. The other zone, the "grabby hands," is a separate element and appears to be the one that directly relates to the relationship. Although I suggested a demon to this patient because of the magnitude of power her boyfriend seemed to be given, she compared his appearance to an alien. Others have represented the many hands as part of a sea creature with claws or pinchers.[7]

Susan Kavaler-Adler examines this territory of codependent relationship and also goes into problems with creativity with her concept of the demon lover complex. Following Fairbairn (1952), she discusses a bad primitive imago or internal object that registers at the magnitude of a demon or "devil" (p. 69). Kavaler-Adler (1993/2013, 1996/2014) describes several characterological manifestations of this relationship and brings in valuable cultural examples from women writers and their "muses." In one note, that is close to my example above, she writes,

> [n]ot only is the power of the woman split off, but the sexual and aggressive impulses that she has trouble containing can also be split off and projected onto the man, lending to the woman an exaggerated form of innocence.
>
> *(Kavaler-Adler, 2010, p. 16)*

As with Rank's nineteenth-century double, Kavaler-Adler writers that "death is the inevitable fate of the woman who is attracted to her demon lover" (ibid., p. 16). Although she has amassed a lot of good material over many books and articles, my hope is to contribute a sophisticated metapsychological model that will allow for more nuanced imago relations to be articulated. Kavaler-Adler conceptualizes the demon lover as being a confluence of the drives of many stages, but some important parameters are missing from her discussions. Projective identification (as a reversal with a parental imago), bad conscience in being treated immorally as one had previously treated others immorally, and specific id impulses aren't brought to bear upon her material.

There is an obvious resonance of the body-based double with the two variations of narcissistic object-choice. Instead of desiring someone who looks like one, shares certain interests, has a similar background, etc., the double looks like and resembles the protagonist. It shows up and either thwarts the protagonist's plans/dreams or enjoys success or romantic conquests in front of him. Instead of a demon lover that relates to the object drives, we have a demon that relates to the ego drives or work relations. Additionally, the double is also linked to bad or "evil," impulses and is readily associated to being a demon that haunts the protagonist or is his "curse." As Rank and Tymms have both indicated, there are further variations of the body-based double than this demon type. However, my interest here is not to be exhaustive in exploring this phenomenon—especially without the full horizontal and vertical axes of the personality being established. I will have to wait until the next book, and the introduction of psychic bisexuality, to venture an adequate conceptualization of the manifest double, the demon lover, and phenomena at this level of development. But, further below I will provide a clinical example of the manifest double to highlight the PI involved.

I would still like to add one more example of a variation of the manifest double in order to show how much interesting material there is for investigation here. Instead of a physical duplicate of one's body, there is a fantasy in which everyone else looks identical except for oneself. For example, in Charlie Kaufmann's *Anomalisa* (2015), the protagonist exists in a world in which everyone looks and talks the same, except for him and a woman he meets, the titular Lisa. The blandness of everyone else and their "land" of bad airplane flights, customer service calls, etc., is an obvious projective identification of the protagonist. Later in the film, as he prepares to make a big speech, the protagonist feels like everything he says is cliché and therefore boring—a moment of inadequacy betrays how he is usually in the place of the interesting parental imago, and projects his self-criticism into both people and the world in which they live. In another variation of this fantasy, *The Matrix Revolutions* (2003) depicts the antagonist, Agent Smith, becoming a virus who has taken over the bodies of everyone within "the matrix" or the computer simulation of earthly reality. The protagonist, Neo, must fight thousands of Agent Smith copies.

In *Willy Wonka and the Chocolate Factory* (1971) and more explicitly in *Charlie and the Chocolate Factory* (2005), the Oompa Loompas are identical little people who live and work in the chocolate factory. Willy Wonka had fired all his human workers after too many of his ideas and recipes were stolen, and the plot of the films is that he opens up his factory for the first time in years, to those who found one of his golden tickets. Wonka creates his own magical world in the factory and with the exception of a human employee, Slugworth (in the first film), he is surrounded by colourful, spontaneous, and magical Oompa Loompas that reflect that world.

Lastly, there is another Charlie Kaufmann film that shows this fantasy and also indicates other important dynamics at this stage of development. In *Being John Malkovich* (1999), there is scene in which all other people look like the actor. Malkovich's uniqueness and celebrity, which the protagonist envies, leads him to try to take over the actor's mind in order to impress a woman. In an interesting scene, the actor himself enters the portal to his own mind, and this results in him seeing everyone present, whether male, female, old, young, etc., as looking like him. The scene does not represent this as being a narcissistic satisfaction, but as a frightening state of affairs. At the end of *Being John Malkovich*, the protagonist is trapped in the mind of the actor but is no longer able to control it. He exists as a consciousness, in the body of another, who must simply behold the external world without being able to have any effect on it. Fantasies of the relation to the mind, control over it, control over another's mind, and the mind being able to leave the body, appear often in clinical work with severe diagnoses. I have had several patients who talk about "astral travel" and leaving their bodies, patients who have talked about ghosts haunting them, and fantasies in which the patient is an animal or can control the mind of an animal. This again points to the importance of Tymms expanding upon the phenomenon of doubling.

I would like to go on to some more formulations of narcissism so that I can get into how Freud includes the double in the larger context of the uncanny. One important formulation concerns the child's "omnipotence," but it is probably more precisely referred to as the egocentrism of the child (Freud, 1914a). For example, Freud (1909b, 1913) found that some patients believed that their wishes or thoughts could magically affect others or the environment (ex. giving someone the evil eye and thinking that this will cause them to mysteriously fall ill or get hit by a car). Freud called this the "omnipotence of wishes" and it is illustrated in our culture in some new age healing practices (ex. Reiki), and positive thinking practices such as The Secret. It is important to know that an individual can have or be attracted to such ideas because they reflect his individual "psychic constitution," and that this is different than the individual who has such ideas because they are considered as true in a group with which he identifies. In some ways, this relates to Freud's point that an obsessional neurosis can be viewed as a "private religion" and that religion is a public neurosis (Freud, 1907, p. 119). So far as an individual believes in a religion, he may have some magical or supernatural beliefs, but he can also say that although he believes in angels, he has never seen one personally. In contrast, an individual without any specific religious affiliations, and no consistent ideology can tell you that he has personally seen an angel or felt its presence in his life.

In general, it is the personal relationship to the supernatural, and magical thinking like the omnipotence of wishes, which takes us to another one of Freud's early conceptualizations of narcissism. Here, the narcissistic is what is outside of "the influence of other people." Freud (1921) writes:

> The contrast between individual psychology and social or group psychology, which at a first glance may seem to be full of significance, loses a great deal of its sharpness when it is examined more closely. It is true that individual psychology is concerned with the individual man and explores the paths by which he seeks to find satisfaction for his instinctual impulses; but *only rarely and under certain exceptional conditions is individual psychology in a position to disregard the relations of this individual to others.* In the individual's mental life someone else is invariably involved, as a model, as an object, as a helper, as an opponent; and so from the very first individual psychology, in this extended but entirely justifiable sense of the words, is at the same time social psychology as well. The relations of an individual to his parents and to his brothers and sisters, to the object of his love, and to his physician—in fact all the relations which have hitherto been the chief subject of psychoanalytic research—may claim to be considered as social phenomena; and in this respect they may *be contrasted with certain other processes, described by us as "narcissistic," in which the satisfaction of the instincts is partially or totally withdrawn from the influence of other people.*
>
> *(p. 69, emphasis added)*

Freud has examples of narcissistic phenomena that are scattered around his work. For example, he views the act of sleep as being a narcissistic retreat from the external world, as a reenactment of the intrauterine environment (Freud, 1917b). Conversely, after the infant leaves the womb, he or she may experience "oceanic oneness" with the external world since the boundaries between it and the ego are at first non-existent and have to be established through successive stages (Freud, 1930, p. 66). The infant is at first an "it" (id) and slowly becomes an "I" (ego) through primary identifications with the caregivers that form the imago, object relations, and the superego (Freud, 1933, p. 64). Freud (1930) writes that narcissistic pathology

> has made us acquainted with a great number of states in which the boundary lines between the ego and the external world become uncertain or in which they are actually drawn incorrectly. There are cases in which parts of a person's own body, even portions of his own mental life—his perceptions, thoughts and feelings—, appear alien to him and as not belonging to his ego; there are other cases in which he ascribes to the external world things that clearly originate in his own ego and that ought to be acknowledged by it. Thus even the feeling of our own ego is subject to disturbances and the boundaries of the ego are not constant.
>
> *(p. 66)*

While it is one thing to project one's sexual desire on to another person, for example, and have the sense that she is being seductive and flirty during mundane conversations, narcissistic phenomena belong to a deeper level. If one projects parts or functions of one's psychic life into the external world, then it can feel like pictures on the walls are listening to one's domestic fights or a cockroach infestation is part of one's bad karma and orchestrated by the universe. If one projects out some aggression and feels a malevolent, ghostly gaze coming from the surrounding environment, for example, hitherto this was only explainable through religious, or superstitious frameworks. Freud does not offer any exhaustive lists of these kinds of narcissistic psychodynamics, but he gives many examples in his essay on "The Uncanny" (1919b). Additionally, along with the narcissistic function of sleep, some disturbances in memory, bodily health, the hunger drive, and other basic functions, can also be shown to be underpinned by psychodynamics related to primitive imagos. The psychosomatic etiology can be elicited from patients in active imagination, in associations from dreams, and other techniques. For example, a patient in a depressed state may describe their body as grey, listless, frozen over, etc. in a fantastical self-observation. With active imagination, for example, she can create a story about a bad witch, a bear with a magical claw, or some fantastical antagonist who cursed or infected a little girl so that she became this grey, listless being. In these fantasies, there are often important bridges to the real-life events (i.e. ego injuries from interpersonal relationships), which led the individual to repress their overwhelming feelings/id impulses and led to defenses being enacted.

Along with active imagination, it is possible to isolate narcissistic phenomena in order to generate ego and object statements. The relation of the individual to the supernatural, his body, inanimate things, animals, psychic functions, etc., can generate such statements that can then be associated to the interpsychic conflicts from which they originated. Here are some examples:

> A female client suffers from an auto-immune problem and has been sick regularly for months. I am impressed with the way she has some splitting with her husband's mother who is seen as a horrible figure who she hates, while her husband is idealized. He would "fight off" his mother and her partner for client, but he is also the reason that they are involved in client's life. She uses the words fight and fighter a few times, and then returns to talk about her auto-immune problems, I interrupt her and ask her to associate to "fighter." Client says "boxer." I ask her to imagine her body is a boxer fighting another boxer representing the viruses that are making her sick and to tell me how she'd describe her body. She says her body is "a sissy, a scared little girl." I ask her to use these as ego statements and see if they feel true for a part of her: "I am a sissy, a scared little girl." Client affirms that it does and I ask her to think who has made her feel like this? She says she can feel this way with her mother-in-law.
>
> A male client fidgets with his work boots and brings up how they are falling apart. He then begins to bring up how he is generally "rough" on his possessions in general. He tells me his car is a mess and is barely reliable and I observe how his clothes are covered with paint, dirt, and have holes in them. I ask him to pretend that the boots he is wearing are a person and for him to try to think about how they might feel about the way he treats them. He gives me statements, "you don't care about me, you don't want to take any time with me, I'm falling apart, I am dying." I ask him to use these as ego and object statements and to see if they feel true about anyone from his past. He tells me that his father comes to mind and that part of him feels like his father didn't show any interest in him when he was younger. He reports that his father worked a lot and that if he spent time with him, that it was in doing the things that his father liked and that his father wouldn't play video, card games, or anything he liked.
>
> A female patient complains of being "institutionalized" and states that she does best when she is told what to do. She brings up the idea that she is "missing part of her brain" and "doesn't know how to do anything on her own" a few times. I ask her to focus on the missing part of her brain and make a few statements about it. I prime her by saying, "you are missing . . . " She says, in an almost exasperated way, "you are not there, you are dead, you are empty." I ask her to say these as object statements and say who comes to mind. She responds that her father does. She goes on to say that if he would have been around when she was younger that she would "know how to handle herself and how to behave" and begins crying as she talks about it.

I ask her what he would have done and she uses general therapy expressions like "give me structure." She opposes this to her mother who she says would ground her, then later ask her to pick up something for her at the store and usually give client money to get something for herself too. With the lack of authority spelled out, and her internal sense for what she needs, I ask her what her father would tell her if he was alive today. She says that he would tell her to "think positively," "encourage [her] to do something," and "be harsh with [her] when [she] need[s] it." This becomes something I use in the transference. I ask her if I should be harsher with her when she misses a session and I ask her if I should be encouraging her to do more as she waits for a call back from her job applications.

A female client gets into "deep sadness" that she expresses as "always wanting love but never being shown love." She first says that she feels it in her chest and then locates the feeling in her heart. She then tells me that it feels like there is a "glass shard in her heart" and I ask her to stay with the feeling there and ask if it feels right to picture a glass shard inside of her heart. I begin BLS and I ask her if the glass shard maps on and she nods that it does. After she signals to me that it's fully embedded she then reports that a "big headache" has come in. I explain to her that this is a block and that her loneliness was probably too big for her to handle. I tell her to stay with the feeling in her head and get more into the feeling of the ache and resume BLS. I then ask her to project it out and she says that she pictures her own head in a vice being squeezed tighter and tighter. Because there is process in the image, I ask her to make a story: if the vice keeps tightening does someone show up to stop it or will something happen to your head? She looks excited and says that her "head explodes" and that she pictures "a big gush of blood and bits of bone come out." I ask her to see if it feels right to picture that gush and bits of bone in her head. She nods after I begin BLS and indicates that it does feel right. I tell her to let it map on to her sensations and let me know when it is fully embedded. She does and I ask if her body or mind has any reaction? She says that "it feels scary to have no head." I ask her if she feels like she is dead and she says no. I wait for her to articulate the feeling and stay silent, but nothing seems to be forthcoming. I ask client to focus on her neck and the rest of her body and to tell me how it feels about missing its head. I begin BLS and she stops me quickly with some fear, and saying that she feels like her neck and shoulders want to "collapse in" and "implode." We discuss whether we should continue with this and she asks to carry on, so I resume BLS. She reports that she has imploded to just her rib cage sticking out of her legs and stomach. She emphasizes with an uncharacteristic tone that she has "no heart and no head." To make sure I understand, I ask more questions and she tells me that she has no arms and is basically just a stomach on legs with no spinal cord. She then clarifies that she has enough of a spine that the bottom of her "boney rib cage" is present.

> I ask her to pay attention to her stomach and the rest of her body and see its reaction to missing her upper body. She says that the remaining part wants the other parts back. I ask her to focus on this desire and see if it is strong enough to regrow the rest. After BLS, she reports that her body grew back to her shoulders, but that her head doesn't regrow. I get the idea to ask her for any words that her body would think about her missing head? I get: "you are gone, lost, broken, damaged." I ask her who comes to mind when she says these as statements about someone she knows or has known. She says that her current boyfriend comes to mind. He is an alcoholic and they have a hot and then cold, he wants her to leave and then wants her to stay, relationship. Despite the mistreatment she gets, she is quick to minimize her beloved's problems or character flaws, and wants to focus on the unity and loving harmony in the relationship (as things had appeared to be at the beginning). I ask her to picture her boyfriend's face when she sees that he is broken, damaged, and lost. She tells me that she "do[esn't] want to believe it." I explain to her that she can't have a head until she sees the deadness in her boyfriend and that part of her already sees this in him. I then empathize that it's awful to recognize that one still feels alone when spending time with a partner. After, she agrees to continue. After the BLS, she reports that her head has regrown after fully seeing his "lostness and brokenness."

In these examples, the narcissistic relations to inanimate things, mental functions, or (parts of) the body are returned to the interpsychic. I introduced the techniques and some of their rationale in the last chapter, and will be introducing some more of the theory involved in Chapters 5 and 6. However, what is important here is that I provide some examples to show that these narcissistic phenomena are still relational and that people have a qualitative sense of such things, even in their relation to inanimate possessions. There are many more examples. I have worked with patients' relationships to the seasons and weather in seasonal affective disorder, to animals, to food, to God, to sleep, to their home, to the world in general, and many more. There will still be examples of some these throughout the book.

The last note I will make on narcissism in this chapter, gets us to a sense of it that is much closer to how it is used today in common language. Narcissistic phenomena in Freud's work is divided between primary and secondary narcissism (1913, 1914a, 1915a, 1919b, 1938a). In the first stage, Freud (1930) differentiates two subtypes: the "man of action" and the intellectual who "seek[s] his main satisfactions in his internal mental processes" (p. 84). Just as there can be survivalist types who aim to be as fully self-sufficient as possible in hunting their own food, fixing all their own machines, etc., there are intellectuals and artists who would rather deal with people through their representations or ideas about them, than actually socializing with them in extended ways. Primary narcissism relates to drives or defenses that see one retreat from social interaction in varying degrees.

This can mean that relations with inanimate things, the environment in general, with supernatural figures or worlds, etc. can begin to take on the energy that normally goes to one's relationships.

In contrast to this introversion of the libido, Freud gives another description of the narcissistic type that can be aligned with the extroversion of secondary narcissism. "People belonging to this type," Freud (1931b) writes,

> impress others as being "personalities"; they are especially suited to act as a support for others, to take on the role of leaders and to give a fresh stimulus to cultural development or to damage the established state of affairs.
>
> *(p. 218)*

Along with this description, Freud comments on their ability to love to emphasize the increase in object relatedness that takes place in later development. The secondary narcissistic individual can be capable of an impressive ability to relate with others, but he or she may be "self-absorbed" and harbor illusions that he is more important, special, or exceptional in society than he really is. The active individual moves from seeming cold and aloof in primary narcissism, to possibly giving the impression of being "cool" and socially desirable in secondary narcissism. In Chapters 5 and 6 I will introduce a more complicated framework that will capture more nuances in the vicissitudes of narcissism.

With this context in place, the central role of Freud's primary narcissistic stages in the uncanny can be appreciated. I will argue that the uncanny is best defined against the encounter with the negative side of the magical, the psychic (in the popular meaning of telepathy, telekinesis, etc.), or some supernatural element that is perceived as a sentient force. In his review of how "uncanny" is commonly used by people (in the German *unheimlich*), Freud (1919b) shows that it is often paired with the eerie, ghostly, horrific, a sense of the gruesome, fear, weirdness, etc. (p. 224). Interestingly, like his research on *mana* and taboo in early cultures, the word *heimlich* (homely) is used in two opposite ways (Freud, 1913). There is the positive sense of feeling close to others, intimate, and comfortable with them, but the term is also used to convey what seems like sarcasm. Doing things that seem like a betrayal of intimacy are also called *heimlich*: talking behind someone's back, having an affair, or other concealed things. "*Unheimlich* is customarily used," Freud reiterates, "as the contrary only of the first signification of '*heimlich*,' and not of the second" (Freud, 1919b, p. 225). Despite his sense that it does not have a relationship to the second sense of the word, Freud does acknowledge Schelling's interpretation, that the uncanny is something that has come to light that should have stayed hidden (ibid., p. 241). In this sense, it may have ties to the other use of homely, because the betrayals of intimacy are often regarded as things that should have stayed hidden as well.

Freud is careful to separate the uncanny from things that belong to the horror genre. In considering how an "unheimlich house" means a haunted house in German, Freud acknowledges the problem of the uncanny being potentially mixed with the "gruesome" or horrific (ibid., p. 241). I take this to mean that the uncanny should not be used to describe a straightforward encounter with evil or the negative side of the supernatural. Instead, the uncanny concerns omens or premonitions of negative supernatural forces. An encounter with a demon in its full physical presence in a horror story, for example, wouldn't be described as uncanny, but signs or evidence that a demon may be behind something that happened would be called uncanny. The state of suspecting that something supernatural is involved, without confirmation, is the first part of the definition of the uncanny; "an uncanny effect is often and easily produced when the distinction between imagination and reality is effaced" (ibid., p. 244). This gives us a formula. First, certain circumstances bring to mind the idea that something may have a supernatural cause, but one still has doubts about whether this could truly be. This also ties to certain operations of the perceptual-consciousness system of the ego that misfire (ex. déjà vu). These problems with ego cognition invoke the sense that something is wrong in the normal or natural order of things, which indirectly points to supernatural forces. Second, if the supernatural element is felt to be negative or dangerous, then the uncanny feeling will continue. If it is a positive supernatural entity, for example, then the story becomes part of fantasy or some similar genre. Third, when the negative supernatural is fully confirmed, then the story moves from the uncanny to the horror genre. For example, it is one thing for children to see a dilapidated and dark house and have the feeling that it might be haunted but if they go inside and have an encounter with a ghost then the story becomes part of the horror genre. However, uncanny elements can still be conserved once the story becomes part of the horror genre. I will return to this shortly.

Along with external supernatural objects, the uncanny can also concern the supernatural in relation to the sense of control of one's own body. This addition to the uncanny encompasses both types of the relation to the double mentioned above. Freud agrees with Ernst Jentsch that observing someone else's seizure or psychotic episode is uncanny because of the "impression of automatic, mechanical processes at work behind the ordinary appearance of mental activity" (ibid., p. 226). In such moments, a non-human force appears to control or possess the person's body or mind. The uncanny effect of hypnotism and diseases that attack cognitive faculties surely fall in this category too. Similarly, instances of seeing someone's multiple personalities take turns controlling her give an uncanny sense that the normal unity of the ego has been overcome. However, some people have the ability to non-consciously imitate the words and mannerisms of others, and there are individuals who can do eerily accurate impressions that can also be uncanny. It's not just the broken mind, but also how the body can become so different in its emotional presence with some people. Freud gives an example of the uncanny feeling in seeing an old man and recognizing that he was looking in the mirror and seeing his own image (ibid., p. 248 fn). He compares this to seeing his double, but since the image wasn't recognized, it seems like the thought would be better captured as the perception that his mind was in the wrong body.

The next stage of the definition of the uncanny concerns how it is conserved in the horror genre. For example, in his discussion of E.T.A. Hoffmann's *The Sandman* (1816), Freud (1919b) writes, "there is no question therefore, of any intellectual uncertainty here . . . and yet this knowledge does not lessen the impression of uncanniness in the least degree" (p. 230). Once a story establishes intellectual certainty of the supernatural, Freud sees the uncanny preserved in two ways. First, uncanniness can reappear through castration anxiety, and second, in the homely returning as a part of the negative supernatural force. Regarding the former, one must understand that castration anxiety takes many forms in psychoanalysis. The idiosyncrasy of literal castration anxiety caught Freud's attention, but in "Inhibitions, Symptom, and Anxiety" (1926a), other important anxiety stages are laid out (ex. birth, loss of the love object, etc.).[8] These stages have different id impulses that issue from body zones. Several different impulses may even share the same zone (ex. spitting, sucking, swallowing, biting, cannibalism, etc., use the mouth). Freud (1919b) draws attention to the fear of the loss of one's eyes, in *The Sandman*, as an example of castration anxiety (p. 231). Another example is the small insect-like aliens in *Alien* (1979), which attach to one's face and then plant eggs in one's body. The hatchlings end up bursting out of one's chest and lead to the death of the host, but having one's face covered, and the sense of something alien living in one's body, are anxiety situations in their own right.

The second way the uncanny is preserved in Hoffman's story, is illustrated in the automaton Olympia, who is a doll brought to life. As a doll, she registers as homely—as something intimate and familiar to one in childhood—and although it is confirmed that a supernatural force gives her life, she is still uncanny. Additionally, even if a supernatural character is on the side of the protagonist and part of the positive supernatural, it can convey an uncanny feeling if it references the homely. However, there needs to be a prominence of the negative supernatural in the story to sustain the uncanny. As mentioned above, seeing a monster, ghost, or demon in its physical form is not uncanny. A traditional demon that is giant, red and has horns, for example, is supposed to inspire great awe and terror. However, a demon possessing a house, and making aspects of it become animated, would conserve the uncanny through the homely. The uncanny exists until the negative supernatural being shows its true form, with one caveat. Sometimes when a demon, or a supernatural creature presents its formerly hidden, full physical form, it possesses certain "homely" human qualities or frailties. For example, the chattering teeth or pins on the head on some of the cenobites (demons) in *Hellraiser* (1987), can leave a lingering uncanny feeling. Similarly, the lack of any visible eyes on the aliens in the *Alien* (1979) and *Aliens* (1986) movies can create an uncanny effect.

These frail or homely aspects of the body of the negative supernatural indirectly relate to castration in its many forms. A body that has lost limbs, has huge wounds/scars, or is missing its eyes, makes id impulses like dismemberment salient to the viewer and conveys an uncanny feeling. However, there is a question of whether this conflates morbid curiosity, or some other lingering attraction to such wounds (or the implements that cause them) with the feeing of the uncanny.

Although Freud (1919b) mentions seeing "dismembered limbs, a severed head, a hand cut off at the wrist" as uncanny, he also adds "feet which dance by themselves" and brings in the supernatural dimension (p. 244). The supernatural, which is formalized in the idea of imagination overtaking reality, is key to the definition. For example, a war movie that depicts a soldier with wounds and missing limbs wouldn't make the film uncanny, although it could certainly make a type of viewer feel uncomfortable or morbidly fascinated. However, I don't want to say that the story must be one that is explicitly supernatural. I am open to the possibility that the camera could linger over the injuries of soldiers in a way that could make a war film feel uncanny. Similarly, there may be intimations that one side of the combatants in the story are inhumanly evil, without this being overt. In such cases the war film would cross genres.

I would like to go beyond Freud's text and discuss a few more elements in the concept of the uncanny. In contrast to the homely in the supernatural, there are certain physical traits that humans may possess that give an uncanny impression because they invoke the supernatural or inanimate. For example, some people have very large, bright doll-like eyes, or very far-away and placid eyes that can induce thoughts of the supernatural. One patient I worked with had a very large mouth with pronounced and curved teeth that often gave me a reverie of a dove or bird flying into the room and the patient catching the bird in her mouth. Alexander Lowen's *The Betrayal of the Body* (1969) shares similar impressions of the physiognomy of certain people. In a truly dialectical psychoanalysis, in which psyche and soma are given equal weight, the body should be seen as an avenue of expression for repression. Additionally, non-universal adaptations, which I will argue for in Chapters 5 and 6, are likely expressed in both body and mind.

Another point concerns an illustration of the uncanny that Freud fails to articulate, and that shows that he was still unsure about some of his formulations. In this example, he writes:

> In the story of "The Ring of Polycrates," the King of Egypt turns away in horror from his host, Polycrates, because he sees that his friend's every wish is at once fulfilled, his every care promptly removed by kindly fate. His host has become "uncanny" to him. His own explanation, that the too fortunate man has to fear the envy of the gods, seems obscure to us; its meaning is veiled in mythological language.
>
> *(Freud, 1919b, p. 239)*

The example of Polycrates resembles the hallucinatory wish fulfillment that Freud attributes to the infant who has its first encounter with the reality principle (Freud, 1911a, 1930). To hallucinate the breast when it is hungry may provide the hungry infant with some momentary contentment, but the emptiness of this hallucination eventually forces an encounter with the reality principle. This principle means that the infant has to separate what is part of its internal Space (i.e. what is imaginary), and what exists in external Space, and will really nourish it. The world of external

Space is created by God/the gods in the fantasy life of humans, and this shows how the reality principle is related to a parental imago whose "prerogative" it is to make something out of nothing (Freud, 1923b, p. 34). For the King of Egypt to see Polycrates conjure up whatever he wants would be uncanny because it resonates with the egocentric wish from his childhood development. Moreover, since it is the prerogative of the gods to create in this way, the king's thoughts go to the envy and wrath of the gods for this insolence, which sustains the uncanny. However, if Polycrates had won his ring from Zeus and knew that he would enjoy Zeus' protection, for example, then it could just be a fantasy or children's story.

Where Freud says that "mythological language" is "obscure" and the meaning is "veiled," I would argue that before psychoanalysis, fable, myth, and other mediums of the supernatural have been the only way to express the magnitude of imago relations. For example, there are many different levels of paranoid jealousy that are visible in the clinic. At the top end, there is jealousy that the beloved might find another man who is more attractive, successful, or "cool" and fall in love with him. Then, there is a person of the upper classes, a celebrity, or a man of higher status of whom to be jealous. Once we go past this point, then mythological language is what gives a sense for the "inhuman" quality of the jealousy. For example, there are many men I have worked with who have many girlfriends or who are having many affairs, but who become very jealous with the thought that one of "their" women might be having a dalliance with another man. This begins to show a part–object relation to women. This kind of person has entered a mythological plane in which he is comparable to a mythological ogre who is terrible and cruel to his harem or severely limits their life. But, this can still go deeper. I have worked with several women who have had jealous boyfriends who locked them in a house and forbade them from spending time with any man, woman, or even a pet. This kind of possessive, jealous person is comparable to a dragon or some creature from mythology that jealously possesses a woman (often with other "treasures") and cares nothing for her desires. She is only allowed to live in her fantasy life or daydreams in its treasure trove.

Lastly, I don't want to privilege the fantasy genre in regards to the uncanny, and it is important to recognize that science fiction, and its roots in technology, also gives us the possibility of non-human sentience that is felt as negative, malevolent, or dangerous. Jentsch's intuition, that a strong theme of the uncanny is inanimate things coming to life, has been recognized by robot designers and those that work with digital special effects in film, under the concept of the uncanny valley (Mori, 2012). In the next book, I will discuss the parallel between the spiritual realms of God-Devil, angel-demon, and magic-black magic, and the "machine." There are fantasies from patients and movies like the *The Matrix* (1999) and the *Terminator* (1984) that make machines into the antagonists. Furthermore, between the horror and sci-fi genres, there is another expression in the concept of negative energy and cursed locations. It's possible that a tree, or some environmental feature, might have a creepy or ominous form and strike a person as uncanny. Although a witch, alien, or non-human creature may be fantasied to be the cause of the negative energy, I have worked with patients who do not invoke either a religious, horror, or sci-fi framework in fantasies. For example, instead of demonic possession or having one's mind controlled by an alien substance, some patients have fantasies of a "black ooze" that makes someone bad. This ooze, for some patients, exists without being put in any larger framework of being from another planet or being demonic. To the extent that the ooze or negative energy is attributed with some awareness or sentience, it should also be included here.

Now that I have formalized some of the implicit ideas in Freud's concept of the uncanny, I'd like to contrast it with the work of a psychoanalytic theorist. Mladen Dolar attempts to tackle the uncanny and the double in "'I Shall Be with You on Your Wedding Night': Lacan and the Uncanny" (1991). As is the case with some Lacanians, he claims that Freud didn't really understand what he had luckily stumbled upon in the concept of the uncanny and is "fortunate that such a paradoxical word existed in the German language" (Dolar, 1991, p. 5). Freud is given respect as the precursor of Lacan, but is also often someone who bungled things, missed the obvious implications of his own work, or was dressed with the flaws of his age—human flaws that Lacan, of course, lacks. Dolar informs us that Lacan created the word extimate (*extimite*) to translate "uncanny" into French and that it gets to the essential dimension of the term:

> It points neither to the interior nor to the exterior, but is located there where the most intimate interiority coincides with the exterior and becomes threatening, provoking horror and anxiety. The extimate is simultaneously the intimate kernel and the foreign body . . . it is this very dimension beyond the division into "psychic" and "real" that deserves to be called the Real in the Lacanian sense.
>
> *(ibid., p. 6)*

Dolar claims that Lacan's object *a* converges with all of the operations of the uncanny/extimate that call into question the status of either the subject or "objective reality." Instead of the sense of the homely, the familiar, or that which belonged to our childhood family life, returning with a negative supernatural aspect, Dolar's use of Lacan's term applies to a very general sense of psychic functioning. Dolar doesn't seek to engage with Freud's analysis, so much as rename things with Lacanian terms. For example, he retraces Freud's analysis of *The Sandman*, and instead of good and bad parental imagos, he mentions the good father of the "universal Law," or the "dead father" of the "name-of-the-father," and the bad father becomes "father-jouissance" who doesn't die and remains a "menacing and jealous figure" (ibid., p. 10). I will engage with the Lacanian concept of jouissance and its ties to the death drive in the next book; I mention it here to show Dolar's approach to overwriting Freud's essay.

When Dolar gets to the analysis of the double, he claims that the good and bad father imago are not in play; these involve a more complicated relation, which becomes a simpler, dyadic relation with the double. The double, like the father-substitute, also dooms the protagonist's efforts to failure, and he acts out the repressed desires that the protagonist's "conscience wouldn't let him do" (ibid., p. 11). In further explanation of the double, Dolar invokes the literal mirror to say that we only have access to the image on the condition of the loss of the object *a*, and that the *a* cannot become an object of knowledge. The operation of the gaze, in his example, means that one can see one's eyes in the mirror but not "the gaze." He adds that if one saw one's image wink, or completely disappear, that this would make the object as gaze appear in the mirror (ibid., p.13).

In contrast to the primary relatedness at the foundation of Freud's model of mind, some Lacanians frequently use paradoxes, or common sense reversals, as a way to keep up a one-person psychology. For Dolar, the double shows up to "spoil and obstruct" the protagonist's desires to win the affection of a woman or get a promotion at work, but only on the surface. In his depth reading, there is a Lacanian reversal in which we should, for example, regard "the magnificent young girl [as] the obstacle to my privileged relation to myself . . . my double" (ibid., p. 14). Dolar's next claim is that truly "join[ing] my real partner, my double . . . [is] joining one's jouissance, [and] regaining one's primordial being, [which] is lethal" (ibid.). He uses Freud's death drive and claims that the double is "protection against 'real death.' It introduces the death drive . . . as a defense against biological death" (ibid.). Dolar doesn't show textual evidence for this in the stories of the double; this interpretation simply exists as a depth reading that stems from his ideological commitments. Closer to the text itself, is not a desire to rejoin one's true partner/double, but the desire to kill the external thing that haunts one. The resulting death of the protagonist by killing his double is more simply explained as projective identification, and the defensive usurpation of the parental imago. Killing the double means that one killed the self imago that has been projected into another (in this case the hallucination of the fantastic double).

I would like to give a clinical example of a patient's manifest double, in order to show that projective identification, and not a relation to one's "primordial being," is what is at stake. A patient's double can sometimes arise from the projection of sensations. Here's an example:

> Client brings up a job he hopes to get and his fear that his criminal record will interfere. He says that he's "scared to hope for it" and that he doesn't "want to be crushed." We discuss the luck involved in this and how someone might see his record and think that it's not worth it, without having any idea of how he's changed or how good he's doing now. He gets into how, when he thinks about this situation, a part of him thinks, "fuck, I'm really trying here" and just wants to "eject" and "give up." Because of the idiosyncrasy of the word eject, I ask him to tell me the first thing that comes to his mind when he thinks of eject, outside of his situation. He tells me that he pictures a "big red button" and that a fist hits it and there's a "meltdown." I ask him to tell me what he sees for this meltdown and he says "everything burns to the ground." I ask him to focus on this picture and tell me if he

has a reaction to it and begin BLS. Likely based upon our previous work, he doesn't give me a bodily zone, but tells me that he's returned to an image that has come up before. He tells me that he sees a "shadowy figure bent over" and this figure shows strong "sadness." I ask him if the image feels different than the last time it came up and he tells me that it's less of a shadow figure and "more of a person . . . and [it] looks like [him]." I ask him if he can keep the image separate from his own feelings or if the fact that it looks like him means that he'll feel like he's talking about himself? Client says he can't keep up the separation, so I ask him to focus on the image and then to describe how he feels. He tells me that he "feel[s] like a total failure" and like he "hates everything and everyone." This part of him feels like he "can't do this anymore" (i.e. keep on the sober path), but, he registers how another part of him "hate[s] that [he] always gives up."

I ask him to stay with these feelings and resume BLS. He tells me that he feels these things in his "gut" and that it's "tied up with thoughts of [him] going to prison . . . [how he] do[es]n't give a fuck about the cops, [his] kids, [his] family." I ask him to stay with the part of him that hates himself for giving up, and how this part wants to stop looking inward and hate everyone on the outside. I ask him to see what he notices and begin BLS. After, he tells me that he judges himself as "worthless, a piece of shit," but then, when he thinks of others who might share this judgment, he thinks "fuck you, look who's talking." I ask him to elaborate and he tells me that it is like he pictures a group of other people, of other addicts, who are "judging [him]" and egg him on by saying, "I told you so, I told you, you'd fail." He says, "fuck you, you're going to fail" as if they are in the office with us. He then says that he has "envy towards them" and wants to ask them "how do you do this [i.e. get high, hurt others, etc.] and never feel bad . . . why do I have a conscience?" I ask him if he's ever seriously wished that he didn't have one and he says yes. I ask him to talk to his conscience, like it was a separate person and see if he can express how he feels about their relationship. He says, "I don't want you, why do you have to interfere, is what I'm doing really so bad, where were you at before I used [before things go bad]?" I ask him to turn these into ego and object statements.

Client tells me that his grandfather comes to mind. I ask him what makes these statements feel true with him and he tells me that his grandfather "is always pestering him." He does a mocking voice and tells me about a time when he was a teen and his grandfather had said, "you're going to regret it [using drugs]." I ask him to focus on these memories of being pestered and see if any one stands out. After BLS, he tells me about one time that his grandfather "knew what was going on" with his drug use, when client had been on probation, and client had told him that he was "going to do what the fuck [he] want[s] to do." I ask client to focus on this memory and see how big his reaction is to it. After BLS, client tells me that he feels a reaction in his chest. I ask him to project it out and he tells me that he pictures a person "with no face." He tells me that he also pictured himself continuing in anger with his grandfather and saying that he's "going to kill people, fuck every bitch, and [that he doesn't] give a fuck." However, right after, he reports that he saw the faceless person "pacing, and worried." I ask client to introject the image and he says it feels right in his chest. I continue BLS and ask him to let me know when it's fully embedded. After he signals me, I ask him to return to the memory with his grandfather and to tell me if it feels differently now. After BLS, he tells me that it felt different and "the way [client] was telling him [his thoughts] was nicer" and there was "more acceptance of what [his grandfather] was going to say." Client looks at me and says his grandfather "was right" and that "he really cared for [client]." I ask client if there's anything we can do with this memory to make it move forward, so he feels closer to his grandfather? He's worked with me for several months and has done this type of reconciliation before and he says yes. I ask him to tell his grandfather what he just told me, and to see if they'll now get along. After BLS, he tells me that he told his grandfather that he "was right, and thank you for always caring and trying to save me." Client continues, "I know you would have [saved me] if you could have" and client adds, "I don't want to go back there [to being rebellious and getting high]." I ask client how it ended and he says that they "hugged" and his grandfather "took it in" and "accepted" him.

I tell client that there's still the issue of the feeling in his stomach and the fire. I ask him to picture "everything burning" and see if he still has a reaction in his gut or in general. After BLS, client reports that he does and I ask him to continue to picture it and see what images come up, or to tell me what gets his focus as he pictures everything burning. After BLS, he tells me that he pictures himself sitting on a chair in a room. I ask him to describe the room and then he strangely tells me that it's not an actual room and that it's "on a mountain," and that he can see his house from the mountain and "[his] whole world . . . [his] house, and everything in [his] life is burning." I ask him to stay with this image and resume BLS. After, he tells me that he has thoughts like "I hate my life, I hate this shit, I hate God." I ask him to focus on his thoughts about God and to elaborate on them. He tells me that "it's like I tried, I tried, and I tried and what the fuck?" "What was the point of all this, to come back to where I am at?" He continues, saying, "I don't understand . . . you made me so special, how come I don't get a family, a wife, and those things . . . how come I don't get those things?" "How come I'm so different than other people?" I ask him what he imagines that God would say back to him and he says, "you're just not ready." He then scoffs, "Fuck, when will I be ready, give me a break!" I try to summarize and say that God seems to be stringing him along but is giving him no guarantees, and client has to see all the good things others get to have in the meanwhile. Client quickly assents and adds that "it's all about faith . . . there's no guarantees." I ask him to say these points as ego and object statements about someone from his past ("you string me along,

> you don't see how hard I've tried, you made me feel special but you don't give me what I want, others get it but not me, you want me to keep waiting but don't give me any guarantees").
>
> Client reports an ex-girlfriend comes up. I ask him to focus on the time when these things felt the truest about her. Client tells me about a time that she kicked him out of the house. He says that "she'd draw [him] in, just enough, but would make [him] keep waiting . . . she'd give no guarantees." He goes on, "this is her way of controlling everything" and then tells me that "no one was better than me at one point . . . then it switched and there was no bigger piece of shit than me." Client talks about helping her with money at that time, how there were likely other guys she was involved with, and there is a low-level anger building as he does. Based upon work with other patients in similar situations, I try to push things forward. I tell client that "her world needs to burn," that the anger he felt towards her was turned on himself, and that he needs to express what he didn't express back then. I ask him to choose a memory that best represents how she treated him and he tells me about a time that she was "swearing at [him], trying to get [him] out of the house, and hitting [him] on the back of the head." I tell him to put himself back in the memory and see what the feeling in his gut wants him to say or do to her. After BLS, client tells me that he "kicked her out of the house" and "took it." He tells me that he called her "a piece of shit" and pointed out how she was "behaving in front of their kids." I ask him what her life is like now that he's in the house and she's out. Client is not sure and so I nudge him and say that I think that her world needs to be in flames. Client looks at me intently and nods and I resume BLS. After, he tells me that he "put her world in flames . . . I put her in the chair" and adds "that's you!" as if she was in the room with us. He adds, "that was never meant to be [him], [he's] not the zero" and "[he] wasn't supposed to be beaten down." I ask him to picture the original memory of her kicking him out and to see if he has a reaction to it, and after BLS he says no. I ask him if he feels anything in his stomach and he says that he doesn't. I ask him if it's just neutral in his stomach or if there's a positive sense of well-being. He says the latter and I ask him to focus on it, and then to float back to another time he felt this well-being there. He tells me that it was when he won an award at school. I ask him to focus on this, where it was, who was around, who he told and as many of the details he can remember. I begin BLS and tell him to let me know when they're in him as much as they can be.

When my patient detailed the relation between him and God and not having the good things that others had, he was explaining how his double wouldn't let him progress in life and have those good things. He was in the place of the castrated parental imago and his double was acting out how he had wanted to light his ex-girlfriend's world on fire, but was doing this to himself. There is an explicit triangulation in his formulations with God, but also an implicit triangulation when one considers the success he's looking for in getting the desired job. There is no primordial being, as Dolar claims, but just aggression towards a parental imago (the ex-girlfriend) that was held back and then a reversal of their places. Similarly, even the bad conscience in my patient's self-hate regarding how he "always gives up" related to his grandfather. It was an intrapsychic tension that came from an interpsychic relation.

In the next part of his article, Dolar wants to put the double in a larger context beyond individual psychology. He seeks to leave the "universal of human experience" and engage with "a specific dimension . . . that emerges with modernity" (Dolar 1991, p. 7). Strangely, he points to ghosts, vampires, and the double as emerging at "a very precise historical moment," as if these things never existed in culture before then (ibid., p. 16). Likely, Dolar is simply talking about the popularity of the romantic and gothic genres at this time, but instead of an explanation for all these supernatural phenomena, we are just given an analysis of Shelley's *Frankenstein* (1822). He sees Shelley's novel as taking up the "limitless possibilities of the new science" (Dolar, 1991, p. 16). The singular or unique monster of Frankenstein does not have a name and cannot be represented by a signifier or be part of the symbolic order (ibid.). Dolar interprets this as being a quest for a "zero degree" of subjectivity that is the missing link between nature and culture: "the point where the spiritual would directly spring from the material" (ibid., p.17). He holds that the monster is excluded from both nature and culture since it isn't allowed to enter the symbolic because Frankenstein will not make him a mate and allow him to found a family.[9] From this Dolar concludes that:

> The paradox of the creature lies in the fact that this embodiment of the subject of enlightenment directly disrupts its universe and produces its limit. The creature, that small extension of scientific endeavor, would fill the missing link and make it exist; it would bridge the gap. With its addition, "the great chain of being" would be complete; one could pass without a break from matter to spirit, from nature to culture . . . but what we would get with this continuous, full universe is the opposite of the traditional *horror vacui*; it is *horror plentitudinis*, the horror of an unsplit world . . . the enlightenment reaches its limit by realizing it.
>
> *(ibid., p. 18)*

Presumably, science ended the previous theological view of the world, and then humans attempt to take on the role of the heavenly Procreator and bridge the gap between Descartes' dualism in the material/body dimension and the "soul" dimension. Instead of recognizing that they cannot create life, Shelley imagines that a human does succeed. Dolar appears to claim that this can't be imagined in a way that is successful and that this failure in imagination—one that creates horrors—is a realization of the limit of science (i.e. it won't allow humans to play God in a happy way). I am sympathetic to this idea, and have had many patients who can't let themselves picture certain behaviors or outcomes in their mind's eye. However,

Dolar goes on to add that "[t]he monster can stand for everything that our culture has to repress—the proletariat, sexuality, other cultures, alternative ways of living, heterogeneity, the Other" (ibid., p. 19). Thus, we move far beyond the specificity of the romantic or gothic period and to the idea that the uncanny "is always at stake in ideology" (ibid.). I won't attempt to evaluate Dolar's claims any further here.

Dolar's analysis of the uncanny returns to the individual level after this, and it is clear that he loses his grasp on Freud's text. First, he quotes Tzvetan Todorov (1973) about the "intellectual uncertainty" involved and compares this to the Lacanian interpretation that he put forward of an "eruption of the real in the midst of familiar reality . . . provok[ing] hesitation and an uncertainty" (Dolar, 1991, p. 21). Dolar invokes this, as if it was not one of the main points of Freud's analysis (Freud 1919b, p. 244). Second, instead of drawing the distinction between the uncanny vs. "the gruesome," or the horror genre, as Freud does, Dolar (1991) claims that even once we are past the uncertainty involved in the uncanny, "the firm knowledge that 'such things don't normally occur' doesn't diminish the uncanny effect" (p. 21). Once the text leaves uncertainty and grants "reality" to the negative supernatural, we saw that the uncanny could persist in relation to the concealment of the bad imago's body, its possession of homely things, or the idiosyncratic form of its attacks or homely body, for example. Dolar does not attempt to show any qualifications or nuances and simply blends the uncanny with horror. Additionally, he tries to express Freud's distinction of imagination vs. reality as the difference between belief vs. knowledge in order to express how we can easily be "duped into anxiety by horror" (ibid.). He contrasts how science is open to doubts and questioning by its nature, but how belief relates to the object *a* and gives a certainty that knowledge will never have. He goes further to say that in the horror genre, "one knows in advance precisely what is bound to happen, and it happens" and that this is "directly opposed to the logic of suspense" (ibid., p. 23). "The fateful events," Dolar writes, "seem unavoidable from the very outset, yet unconsciously one doesn't believe that the unavoidable will happen" (ibid.). He continues:

> [T]here is a passage from "I know very well . . . yet I believe" to "I don't really believe . . . yet I am certain." The mechanism of uncanniness doesn't leave you any space for uncertainty and hesitation. If there is a structural hesitation, or floating, attached to it, it comes from the impossibility of espousing the terrible certainty . . . From a Lacanian perspective the uncanny comes from too much certainty, when escape through hesitation is no longer possible, when the object comes too close.
>
> *(ibid.)*

Dolar's very general account of the uncanny, which involves the structure of belief itself, is a Lacanian reversal of the willing suspension of disbelief. In the latter, one knows "very well" that one is watching a horror movie and can consciously think about the generic conventions of the story that are unfolding but still find oneself caught up in the anxiety situations. As I understand him, Dolar's reversal is to say that the unconscious knows (with certainty) that there will be a terrible encounter with the anxiety object, and the ego's position is to vicariously doubt the reality of the supernatural. Primary engagement with the text is not on the level of the generic conventions but on the level of the unconscious, with the doubting ego being forced into anxiety when the terrible situation or object "comes too close." In this way, one is not primarily a rational spectator, but engages in identification with the characters first, and with the ego trying to talk oneself down from the vicarious certainty of the frightening antagonists that map onto one's own bad imagos. While I do agree with the idea of primary engagement with a story through emotional identification, Dolar's formulation can be applied to all genres, and therefore does not give us an insight into the uncanny. For example, in watching a James Bond movie, one could similarly feel like Bond could lose in a fight scene or be killed when captured by the villain. However, a story can involve the threat of death or some other anxiety situation, but not be uncanny. The very general concept of the object *a* isn't capable of giving a nuanced account, or if it is, Dolar does not get much out of it.

Notes

1 This idea of death relating to a later stage of development while early destructiveness cannot be held to have this aim, has found articulation before. For example, Winnicott (1960) writes: "[a]nxiety in these early stages of the parent-infant relationship relates to the threat of annihilation . . . '[I]nherited potential' is becoming itself a 'continuity of being'[;] [t]he alternative to being is reacting, and reacting interrupts being and annihilates. Being and annihilation are the two alternatives . . . At this stage the word death has no possible application, and this makes the term death instinct unacceptable in describing the root of destructiveness. Death has no meaning until the arrival of hate and of the concept of the whole human person. When a whole human person can be hated, death has meaning, and close on this follows that which can be called maiming; the whole hated and loved person is kept alive by being castrated or otherwise maimed instead of killed. These ideas belong to a phase later than that characterized by dependence on the holding environment" (p. 591).

2 Freud (1914a) also has a (c) and a (d) but it is a stretch to see how they relate to finding the self in the desire for the object. He writes, "(c) what he himself would like to be, (d) someone who was once part of himself," and although there may be an insight here that I can't grasp, what is striking about narcissistic object-choice is the great many similarities a person shares with the love object (p. 90). To take just one trait or their occupation, for example, loses the magnitude of the desire.

3 We saw that the literal mirror was not important for psychosexual development, but narcissistic object-choice, sexual fascination with one's own body, discomfort with seeing one's mirror image, etc., are real clinical phenomena. Once we see that socioeconomic issues enter narcissistic object-choice, the issue of the child not recognizing its mirror image is the least worry for someone who is using an atomistic model of the individual. It would be "adultomorphic" to say that the pre-verbal child somehow comprehended aspects of its socioeconomic class and the traits of identity that are present in examples of narcissistic object-choice. Instead, what is at stake is a relation of difference between the self imago and the parental imago that allows for one's identity to be conceptualized through physical appearance, on one hand, and basic taxonomic or classifying acts of perception, on the other. Once language is learned, it has to be connected with these pre-linguistic acts of taxonomy—acts that both children and animals observably perform

in interaction with their environment. In other words, the cognition involved in early acts of perception do not involve things like socioeconomic class at the time that this cognitive faculty is formed, but when the child develops more object relatedness, which will later be transcribed to the social body, the same simple acts of perception are needed to recognize classifications there. A discussion of the development of cognition in the work of Kant and Hegel will be offered in the next book.

4 This form of narcissistic object-choice resembles Rank's insight that "a man's past—represented in the film by the hero's own youthful image—is so intimately bound to his vital being that misfortune befalls him if he tries to detach himself too completely from it (Rank, 1941, p. 69). The double often appears as possessing the brazen and confident youth that a protagonist no longer has, and the partners of these women, in some cases, similarly represent the selfish and immature youth that they had disowned.

5 In *The Economics of Libido* (2015) I argue that the classical contrast between the narcissist and masochist in psychoanalysis often represents the passive-masochist as an inverted narcissist and the altruistic drives as reaction formations against sadism. Following Freud's (1913, 1917c) recognition of separate egoistic and altruistic drives, the recognition of reparation coming from the life drives in Klein (1975), and analysts like Eigen (1986) who argue for separate poles that combine in dialectical syntheses, I saw a need to rename the binary of narcissism and masochism. Although I was unaware of his use of it at the time, I agree with Davis (2005) that echoism is the most salient term. I will revisit this binary again in the next book, when I re-introduce psychic bisexuality, but I would like to make a quick note here. For many echoists, the primitive suppression of aggression is so severe that when anger, hate, etc. is called up in them by extreme mistreatment, they are unable to express it even in fantasying. They will say that they feel impotent; the other person they feel the aggression towards feels too powerful, they feel too small, etc. However, they sometimes are able to express, and process, the destructiveness vicariously through an animal who attacks the person in their fantasy.

6 As with most clinical advances, I know to introduce these ideas and be more active because previous patients, with whom I had been more passive, produced this material themselves. When I see someone is representing a bad figure in his or her life as unrealistically powerful and entering a supernatural level, I will suggest different magnitudes of power such as evil mastermind, demon, the devil, etc. and try to help the patient articulate the felt magnitude of the imago in question. Similarly, I have found that using terms like king or queen, when discussing a person's sense of how powerful they viewed themselves to be in the past often resonates and produces more expressive communication about individual narcissistic states.

7 In therapy, there are variations outside of the demon with many grabby hands, or claws or pinchers (as other patients have described it). Others have projected out demons and introjected them from their chest and shoulders. Some have projected winged demons and introjected the wings in their backs. Additionally, it is a very uncanny experience for them to be engaging in fantasying in therapy and share how they cannot imagine, or let themselves picture certain outcomes with a demon. For example, one patient imagined he was in a neighborhood and trying to find his way home but a demon would show up to block him from getting to his house. No matter what he tried in his fantasy, the demon always showed up to stop him and he stopped the fantasying with a massive sense of futility.

8 Analogously, sex becomes Eros in Freud's work and a synonym for human connection or social energy in which sex is one relation and romantic love, familial love, friendship, etc. are other expressions (Freud, 1920, p. 50).

9 There is a parallel between my patient's frustration with God for not allowing him to have a wife and family and what Dolar points to in Frankenstein's monster being barred from the symbolic because he isn't given a mate to create a family, nor a name. However, I cannot accept the idea that the contingent, symbolic dimension in Lacan's work is what is responsible for establishing the salience of someone's name nor her recognition of her own

mirror image. First, there are animals that pass the mirror test, which shows that language is not needed. Second, increasing object relatedness, which drives one to care for others, is a necessary reference point as the motivation to want to use language in order to inquire about them, know their whereabouts, or want to tell stories about them. Third, a developing mimetic sense, which allows one to recognize one's own bodily movement in the mirror, is another necessary reference. If one can recognize one's own mirror image without language, then mimetic cognition and increasing object relatedness can also be the basis of differentiating oneself from others in order to make use of the language game of naming.

3

THE LATENT AND PATRIARCHAL DOUBLE

The latent double

In contrast to the manifest double, there are no longer any ties between a double and the body or blood of the protagonist with the latent double. Instead, the second school looks for hints of shared identity, places an emphasis on moral opposition or the complementarity of characters, an idiosyncratic and unmotivated change in a character, etc., to argue that one or more characters are covertly doubled in a text. Once we enter this territory, it becomes clear that not every author could have self-consciously chosen to double their characters. However, there are may be many self-conscious reasons for an author to use the manifest, supernatural double in a story: the fashion of a given period or an author choosing to imitate another writer.

Additionally, as critics like Webber (1996), Herdman (1990), or Miyoshi (1969) posit, the double is an attractive device for an artist to express philosophical or religious ideas, or be an extension of/react against previous genre conventions. It is also possible that an author might claim that he had a conscious intention to use the double, but this could be a secondary elaboration or rationalization, when he was really drawn to it because of how it resonated with his own primary narcissistic fantasies. However, where critics of psychoanalysis can give other reasons for the creation or use of the manifest double, it is difficult to see how they could claim that every author had intended to use latent doublings in their narratives. Part of the reason that I include a film like *The Lost Boys* (1987) in this book is because the writers and filmmakers of this, and similar fare in popular culture, could not be accused of being intellectuals who purposefully apply psychoanalytic ideas.

Freud's commentary on Lady Macbeth in Shakespeare's famous play, mentioned in the introduction, and credited by him to Ludwig Jekels, is the first example of latent doubling. It bears being quoted again:

> [W]ith Macbeth and Lady Macbeth . . . it would of course be pointless to regard her as an independent character and seek to discover the motives for her change [;] . . . the germs of fear which break out in Macbeth on the night of the murder do not develop further in *him* but in *her*. It is he who has the hallucination of the dagger before the crime; but it is she who afterwards falls ill of a mental disorder. It is he who after the murder hears the cry in the house: "Sleep no more! Macbeth does murder sleep . . ." and so "Macbeth shall sleep no more"; but we never hear that *he* slept no more, while the Queen, as we see, rises from her bed and, talking in her sleep, betrays her guilt. It is he who stands helpless with bloody hands, lamenting that "all great Neptune's ocean" will not wash them clean, while she comforts him: "A little water clears us of this deed"; but later it is she who washes her hands for a quarter of an hour and cannot get rid of the bloodstains: "All the perfumes of Arabia will not sweeten this little hand." Thus what he feared in his pangs of conscience is fulfilled in her; she becomes all remorse and he all defiance. Together they exhaust the possibilities of reaction to the crime, like two disunited parts of a single psychical individuality, and it may be that they are both copied from a single prototype.
>
> *(Freud, 1916, pp. 323–324)*

The relation of Lady Macbeth to Macbeth compares to some of Freud's remarks in "The Uncanny" (1919b). In the story of *The Sandman* (1816), he uses another term, "dissociated complex," to refer to Olympia's relation to Nathaniel (Freud, 1919b, p. 232). Freud holds that she betrays Nathaniel's "feminine attitude" towards his father and that his "senseless, obsessive love for Olympia" is explained as narcissistic love (ibid.). As mentioned in the last chapter, instead of falling in love with someone who physically and/or psychically resembles oneself, the other type of narcissistic object-choice concerns how the beloved represents what one used to be. He or she can embody a dissociated aspect of one's personality, along the horizontal axis of psychic bisexuality, and in some cases, represent his whole active or passive pole. The latent double of the protagonist follows this version of narcissistic object-choice, as long as long as one recognizes that the ego drives take objects as well. Additionally, the reaction of bad conscience and a subsequent symptom, as in Freud's example above, is another variation of this. The rest of the writers considered within this part of the literature review follow Freud in looking for "disunited parts" of both protagonist and antagonist, without the fantastical, body-based ties of the first school.

Robert Rogers, in *A Psychoanalytic Study of the Double in Literature* (1970), coins the distinction between the manifest vs. latent double that I have used in this chapter. In his view, the latter primarily concerns how one character can be a foil of another and represent his or her "conflicting drives, orientations, or attitudes" (ibid., p. 5). If the latent double displays these drives, orientations, and attitudes in relation to other characters in the text, then this is *object doubling*, if he or she simply represents the antithetical, then it is an example of *subject doubling*. This division is also made according to whether the doubled character is related to the protagonist or not. For example, in Dostoevsky's *The Brothers Karamazov* (1880), Father Zosima is both a foil to the lecherous father Karamazov and a parental/authority figure. Additionally, Rogers interprets *David Copperfield* (1850) as having a "veritable galaxy of father, mother, and wife figures" (Rogers, 1970, p. 115). Along with all these doubles among the parental-substitutes, Uriah Heep is very much a complementary latent double to the titular character, and Rogers points out his shared identity with David Copperfield in how "he too reaches adolescence and maturity without the assistance of a father" (ibid., p. 115). Rogers' procedure for the identification of doubles is very open-ended. This is both a strength and a weakness, as I will show below.

Rogers hypothesizes a psychological cause for doubling in his assertion that "mental conflict within a single mind" is most naturally dramatized "by two or more characters" (ibid., p. 29). In doing so, he holds that "[s]urreptitious doubling allows for a relatively uninhibited, anxiety-free identification of the reader with the protagonist, an identification made possible by the displacement of the hero's guilt onto his secret sharer" (ibid., p. 58). As mentioned in the Introduction, his hypothesis of an anxiety-free identification with the protagonist is similar to, and antedates, my thoughts about what was going on in *The Lost Boys*. I would add that beyond anxiety there is also unpleasure, superego tensions, and other intrapsychic conflicts that may be potential causes of doubling, but these are small points to add to Rogers' insight.

Rogers' main way of identifying latent doubles is by the "complementarity of personality traits" (ibid., p. 23). An example of this complementarity is how a protagonist's idealistic attitudes towards women may be doubled in another character he sees as a "lecher" (ibid., p. 35). This leads Rogers to acknowledge that

> [a]n almost ineluctable dualism would seem to haunt our categories of the double in literature. Masochist and Sadist, Loyal son and Rebellious son, Loved Father and Hated Father, Pure Mother and Mother-as-Whore, Fair Maid and Femme Fatale—they sound so polarized that skeptics might accuse the psychoanalytic critic of perpetrating a hideous and intolerable system of allegory instead of doing his job with at least a semblance of scientific rigor.
> *(ibid., p. 138)*

Rogers goes on to argue for the merits of allegory, and descry its unfashionable status in English Departments. He cites Freud's "A Seventeenth-Century Demonological Neurosis" (1923a) as recognizing that religious thought would conceptualize the neurosis of its day in allegory involving demons, possession, or trafficking with the devil. Along with complementarity, Rogers chooses some texts in which narrators make explicit references to a second character as a secret sharer or other self. As illustrated in films like *Psycho* (1960) and *Fight Club* (1999), there can be an introspective awareness of the latent double so that the author may reveal it to be non-existent in a twist ending. Comparably, an author can become aware that she has created a latent double and consciously add ties between it and the primary character or, as mentioned above, she may have self-consciously set out to create a latent double in imitation or paying homage to this form in the work of another writer. Lastly, Rogers (1970) mentions "structural considerations," such as two characters being together at the beginning or the end of a story, as an important hint of their shared identity (p. 46). In stories with many potential doubles, I have found this structural bookending to be particularly helpful.

Rogers makes several small, but important differentiations when he considers the psychoanalytic roots of latent doubling. He employs the technical term *decomposition* as the opposite to condensation. In the latter, a thing in a dream represents more than one event, person, or relation, while the former is the process in which different aspects of the same person are represented by different people. Rogers does not match the mechanism of decomposition to any psychosexual stage, nor does he identify the projective identification that can often be involved; he admits that "most of the time the psychosexual genesis of doubling lies so deeply buried that only profound analysis will unearth it" (ibid., p. 16). Like Rank, he interrogates the myth of Narcissus and emphasizes that the narcissist's self-love does not preclude that he takes lovers. Rather, narcissism can be expressed through how a person is merely interested in sex and is unable to love, because ideals like permanent youth, beauty, or superlative success are valorized. Lastly, Rogers also agrees with Rank that the double can be a conscience or superego figure. However, he does not offer any discussion of different types of conscience, nor how the superego functions in early stages of development, so this remains rather opaque in his study. Rogers has many solid intuitions, and made the greatest advancements in the second school of double scholarship, but lacks a psychoanalytic model of personality that is sophisticated enough to formalize them.

In "The Idea of the Double" (1978), Doris Eder is critical of what she sees as Roger's doubling mania. Although she recognizes that his work is more "penetrating" than that of other critics, she also asks how identifying so many doubles in a single work has illuminated anything in the story (ibid., p. 589). While examples like Lady Macbeth serving as a double for Macbeth's guilt and general complementarity help the psychologically minded reader appreciate a character more fully, I agree with Eder. Doubling in the second school of scholarship can appear as an end in itself, and as one that detracts from the overall plot or story. In the symptom reading, I will show how doubling is performed in the service of the plot, even though complementarity, or other principles, might suggest that more doubles exist in the story.

Interestingly, Eder (1978) registers a literary movement that goes beyond the principal of complementarity in the second school to a new type of double in the work of Herman Hesse and modernist authors. This new definition of the double sees dualism as too simple, thus valorizing further complexity or multiplicity. She also registers the "self-consciousness" of the writers in modernism, noting how the multiple personalities are employed stylistically (ibid., p. 613). While this may represent a legitimate phenomenon in literature, it is difficult to see how it escapes her own criticism of Rogers' doubling mania, and it is outside of my interest to investigate it further. Such authors may have had a stylistic interest in showcasing the complexity of their internal world, and perhaps this came from knowledge of psychoanalysis, but Eder does not make the significance of this clear.

In *The Literature of the Second Self* (1972), Keppler attempts to differentiate himself from others who have studied the double by focusing on what he calls *the second self*. As opposed to manifest doubling, he wants to focus on how

> [t]he first self is the one who tends to be in the foreground of the reader's attention, usually the one whose viewpoint the reader shares; he is the relatively naïve self, naïve at least in tending to suppose that he is the whole self, for he seldom has any conscious knowledge, until it is forced upon him, of any other self involved in his make-up. The second self is the intruder from the background of shadows, and however prominent he may become he always tends to remain half-shadowed; he is much more likely to have knowledge of his foreground counterpart than the latter of him, but the exact extent and source of his knowledge, like the exact nature of his motivation, are always left in comparative obscurity.
>
> *(Keppler, 1972, p. 3)*

For Keppler, the objective second self (duplication in body) and the subjective one (duplication of an unconscious aspect of the personality) are often too easily read as part of the protagonist's psychology. He believes it is problematic for the reader or critic to be quick to regard both of them as having no real existence in the story. Towards this end, he makes it a point to exclude examples of physical duplication through a shadow, mirror image, statue, portrait, etc. unless it becomes a living personality that has a "counterbalancing" relationship with the protagonist (ibid., p. 7). Furthermore, Keppler gives the example of Poe's *William Wilson* (1839) in which physical duplication is also a symbol of an "internal continuity" and "deeper bond" (Keppler, 1972, p. 7) as a true second self. On the subjective side, he notes that in cases of a split personality the second self does not achieve its own independent existence. For example, in Stevenson's *Strange Case of Dr. Jekyll and Mr. Hyde* (1886), Mr. Hyde does not confront Dr. Jekyll; while one personality is dominate, the other lies in a trance-like state. Along with this example, Keppler excludes different forms of possession, changes in personality wrought by hypnotism, and allegorical forms of literature that personify traits like envy or greed. Again, the second self can be drawn from either the objective or subjective types, but must be "a self in his own right" but with his "psyche intergrown by untraceable shared tendrils with that of his counterpart" (Keppler, 1972, p. 10).

Keppler lists many ways in which these tendrils with the second self may show up. He cites how the intrusion of the second self into the life of the first self can never be entirely accounted for by logical reasoning. He points to the affinity between the two selves as shown in inexplicable emotional reactions, whether in antagonism or attraction, or by an intimate insight into the mind of the other (usually the double's insight into the protagonist). He also discusses how the second self can be referred to as the self that has been excluded from the first self's sense of his own identity (i.e. the first self refers to the second as his opposite or he can be viewed as complementary to him). Keppler does not try to investigate whether the author had the conscious intention to create a second self. Instead he compares the creation of both to the fantasy that underlies a child's make-believe friend, as well as the more unconscious processes that form the symptom of a mental disorder.

Keppler speculates about the psychological cause of the double not through psychoanalytic stages, but through a more philosophical sense of time. "More readily imaginable," he writes, "is the second self who represents a certain stage of development . . . *within* the first self's own lifetime" (ibid., p. 172). He reasons that the double could represent a stage not yet reached, but one that is anticipated, or a stage the first self has already experienced and of which the second self is a memory. However, Keppler does not go on to offer a developmental theory, nor does he go into existing psychoanalytic theory to give a foundation to this hypothesis. Instead, he considers his work "the preliminary" to any such answer (ibid., p. 182). He acknowledges that Rogers' manifest vs. latent double is similar to the objective and subjective category that he outlines, but is critical of Rogers for not observing that the two categories can be mixed, as in the case of Poe's *William Wilson*. Along with this uncharitable reading, Keppler also believes that Rogers' work is not a true investigation, but rather a demonstration of "an already established doctrine regarding the nature of the human psyche" (ibid., p. 186). Oddly, he writes this as if Rogers simply looked into a dictionary of psychoanalysis, found the relevant entry, and applied the ideas without seeing what was suggested in the texts themselves. Psychoanalytic theory has many schools and is far from an established doctrine. Being able to argue that a given narrative more closely resembles one psychodynamic process than another is valuable in such a state of pluralism. Moreover, it is very confusing to see how his "preliminary" work is supposed to lead to the creation of a wholly new model of the mind that does not reference a model that is derived from those doing clinical work. Lastly, his hypothesis seems derivative of Rank's idea "that misfortune befalls [one] if he tries to detach himself too completely from [his youthful image]" (Rank, 1941, p. 69). Hostility towards psychoanalysis seems to define his interpretative stance more than having found a different or better way in which to make sense of the latent double.

Margaret Tarratt's "Monsters from the Id" (1986) does not explicitly reference the double, as the other works in this section do, but it follows Freud's idea of one character representing something dissociated from another character. Because she provides a procedure for interpretation, I will spend a bit more time summarizing one of the films in her article. Tarratt begins by indicating that although several commentators assert that the romantic subplot in science fiction narratives is forced or unnecessary, she believes that it is "an integral part of their structure" (ibid., p. 260). Conflicts with aliens or monsters are held to be an externalization of the protagonist's battle with his own sexual desires: desires that cannot be expressed in a romantic subplot. Tarratt holds that this externalization is caused by the protagonist's "sexual animal" desires coming into conflict with his social being, which is influenced by "civilized" morality.

In her analyses, Tarratt establishes relevant symbols of sexual desire within the narrative. For example, in the film *The Thing (from Another World)* (1951), she shows a parallel between the scientists discovering that the alien Thing's hand is its sexual organ, and how the protagonist, Captain Hendry, expresses his sexuality through his hands, exemplified in his desire to touch Nikki, his love interest. Nikki binds Hendry's hands in order to feel safe when meeting him, and he later receives an injury to one of his hands that she nurses. These events allow her to find him "acceptable" because of the "forcible taming of his aggressive sexuality that civilized society demands" (Tarrat, 1986, p. 266). Tarratt writes that, "the manner in which he handles the military situation created by the Thing's presence is an image of the way in which he handles himself in relation to Nikki" (ibid., p. 267). She also intuits a parallel between the frozen environment in which the military discovers the Thing and the repressed emotional and sexual life of the all-male expedition before the group of airmen and Nikki arrive.

Tarratt has a convincing confidence in her analysis when she states, "the Thing clearly represents Hendry's repressed sexual desires, the impulses of the id" and concludes by writing, "the structure of this film can only be understood in a Freudian context" (ibid., p. 266). Out of all the works on the double, her way of interrogating the text resonated most with me. However, there are three issues with Tarratt's approach. First, Tarratt seems to unnecessarily reduce herself to "id sexuality" instead of being open to the possibility of an interpsychic model of the monster and its relation to others. The fear that the men in the film feel towards the monster, may be read as the fear of Nikki towards Hendry, for example. This is not to say that one cannot examine things from this side of a person struggling with his own desires, but I will show how both sides of the ego–object relation are manifest in the symptom reading. The second issue is that Tarratt's analysis is confined to the realm of the fantastic (i.e. sci-fi, horror, etc.). Fantastical beings are what first gave me the idea for a symptom reading too, but the double criticism of the second school shows that one can perform such readings with non-fantastical beings too. The third issue is that non-Freudian critics have had similar intuitions about doubling, and ideas about pathetic fallacy, for example, existed long before psychoanalysis. In this way, Tarratt overstates her case when she writes that psychoanalysis provides the only way to understand the structure.

What is specifically psychoanalytic, and not merely intuition, requires a reference to metapsychological concepts—concepts that have had very little growth in psychoanalysis since the 1940s. An imago from psychosexual development will be connected to different types of ego cognition. These forms of ego cognition go along with personality disorders such as the impressionistic cognition of the histrionic personality or different forms of compulsion in the obsessional personality (Shapiro, 1999). Every imago has a different form of id aggression and affection, such as impulses to cannibalize, to behead, to dismember, to be embraced, to be given a baby, to be in someone's loving gaze, etc. Then there are bodily zones related to these id drives, which go far beyond the oral, anal, and phallic. The hand, the shoulders, the head, the eyes, the stomach, the tongue, and many more zones are salient in clinical work. Lastly, these all have to be plotted on the horizontal axis of psychic bisexuality and the vertical axis of the superego development. My hope is that this book will contribute to the resurgence of metapsychology.

The double of patriarchy

The third school of the double emerges from the seminal text of Gilbert and Gubar, *The Madwoman in the Attic* (1979). This school references the touchstone of patriarchy and limiting gender roles, with individual psychology taking a backseat, if it is given any credit at all. Gilbert and Gubar hold that female characters in nineteenth-century literature are represented as either angelic and good, or rebellious madwomen. The female writers of the time are seen as lacking role models outside of these gender roles and Gilbert and Gubar interpret doubling as a subtext to deal with this lack. The doubles, which they name *avatars*, are viewed as the by-product of how female writers struggled to define new roles that went beyond gender dichotomies. They write:

> Images of enclosure and escape, fantasies in which maddened doubles functioned as asocial surrogates for docile selves, metaphors of physical discomfort manifested in frozen landscapes and fiery interiors—such patterns recurred throughout this tradition, along with obsessive depictions of diseases like anorexia, agoraphobia, and claustrophobia.
>
> *(ibid., p. xi)*

Although Gilbert and Gubar observe how mental pathology is caught up with other fantasies in the text, they choose to sociologically interpret the cause of their appearance in the oppression of women. It is possible to look at the psychological causes of these mental illnesses and link them to problems of specific psychological types, which can be studied in the texts, but Gilbert and Gubar go on to judge that the

> artists we studied were literally and figuratively confined . . . for not only did a nineteenth-century woman writer have to inhabit ancestral mansions (or cottages) owned and built by men, she was also constricted by the Palaces of Art and Houses of Fiction male writers authored. We decided, therefore, that the striking coherence we noticed in literature by women could be explained by a common, female impulse to struggle free from social and literary confinement through strategic redefinitions of self, art, and society.
>
> *(ibid., pp. xi–i)*

Despite these claims of the importance of culturally prescribed limitations, when the authors move into textual analysis, they do so "on a figurative and psychological level" (ibid., p. 359). For example, in regards to *Jane Eyre* (1847), Gilbert and Gubar (1979) hold that

> what Bertha now *does*, for instance, is what Jane Eyre wants to do. Disliking the "vapour veil" of Jane Rochester, Jane Eyre secretly wants to tear the garments up. Bertha does that for her too. Resenting the new mastery of Rochester, whom she sees as "*dread* but adored" (ital. ours), she wishes to be his equal in size and strength, so that she can battle him in the contest of their marriage. Bertha, "a big woman, in stature almost equaling her husband," has the necessary "virile force" (Chap. 26). Bertha, in other words, is Jane's truest and darkest double: she is the angry aspect of the orphan child, the ferocious secret self Jane has been trying to repress ever since her days at Gateshead. For, as Claire Rosenfeld points out, "the novelist who consciously or unconsciously exploits psychological Doubles" frequently juxtaposes "two characters, the one representing the socially acceptable or conventional personality, the other externalizing the free, uninhibited, often criminal self."
>
> *(ibid., pp. 359–360)*

Women of the nineteenth century undoubtedly faced patriarchal restrictions, and, in some cases, this may have been the cause of repression of parts of their personality. Bertha's size and uninhibited anger suggests a narcissistic superiority that is a part of Jane and reacts to the unequal marriage arrangement that Rochester is offering. Jane and Rochester both felt an equality that attracted them to one another, but Rochester does not act from the part of him that feels this, and Jane experiences rage in seeing him take advantage of his male privilege. Bertha ultimately burns down Rochester's home and Gilbert and Gubar do an excellent job in showing how her actions can be attributed to feelings and motivations that are intimated in Jane's character. It is only when Rochester has suffered this loss, is physically reduced in power, and Jane receives an inheritance that raises her social level, that she returns to marry him. These aspects of the repressed/dissociated parts of power/narcissism in Jane's character can further be studied in the repetitions and defenses that are evident in her relation with Rochester.[1]

My issue with this approach to doubling is that Gilbert and Gubar reference psychology in analyzing the protagonist's latent double, but drop all references to it once they discuss the female author's "anxieties of authorship" and the gender roles with which she is confronted. A priori, they claim the problem is "based on the woman's socially determined sense of her own biology" and do not offer arguments for this view or against individual psychology (ibid., p. 51). They write:

> The loneliness of the female artist, her feelings of alienation from male predecessors coupled with her need for sisterly precursors and successors, her urgent sense of her need for a female audience together with her fear of the antagonism of male readers, her culturally conditioned timidity about self-dramatization, her dread of the patriarchal authority of art, her anxiety about the impropriety of female invention—all these phenomena of "inferiorization" make the woman writer's struggle for artistic self-definition and differentiate her efforts at self-creation from those of her male counterpart.
>
> *(ibid., p. 50)*

There are no arguments for the "culturally conditioned" aspects of the female author's personality. As mentioned above, there are cases in which the discipline and punishment that sometimes enforces social norms can lead to the suppression of parts of the personality that are deemed antisocial. However, this is not the sole cause of repression, and there are psychosexual causes of timidity in the passive pole in the personality. Additionally, there were also many women who were in touch with their active pole and were in possession of power and confidence, even though they were barred from many institutions in society. Gilbert and Gubar's universalization of female experience is overly simplistic, open to many counterfactuals, and based upon a social constructivism that breaks down in simple interrogations.

I agree that gender can have an influence on someone's personality, but it is not the sole cause nor is it impossible to differentiate the psychological and sociological inputs. For example, after receiving ego injuries, both women and men can have ego identifications that can see them limit themselves to gender roles. Such identifications are analogous to identification with the aggressor, or Stockholm syndrome, in which the aggressed party takes on the point of view of the aggressors. For example, a girl in middle school can be bullied or shamed in regards to her lack of attractiveness, cheap clothing, etc., and react by internalizing the standard of beauty, or sharing the same cultural ideal with the bullies. However, not all women try to change their body type or dress in competition to best approximate a cultural ideal of beauty. Similarly, not all creative women are "timid about self-dramatization," and the psychology Gilbert and Gubar employ in their readings of novels is thrown out for the easy answer of "cultural conditioning."

The claim that the female anxiety of authorship is "a radical fear that she cannot create, that because she can never become a 'precursor' the act of writing will isolate or destroy her," is very strong language (ibid., p. 48). Any good clinician knows to pay attention to such language because it has ties to early imago relations. "Radical fear," "dread," and "being destroyed," in Gilbert and Gubar's passage are commensurate with infantile feelings and infantile estimates of the power of parental imagos. Their language likely references something in *their* psychology (i.e. their issues with individual assertiveness, for example) more than something universal in the experience of women. In contrast, when ego identifications involving gender roles are in evidence, what is the most salient is how closed off the person is about entertaining options outside of the stereotypical. For example, there are some men who, beyond individual appreciation of things like sports, hunting, fishing, trucks, etc., think all other men should be interested in them too, and who don't like to hear any disparaging remarks about their interests. There is a frozen, rigid take on "manliness" and if such a man comes in with anxiety issues, for example, he can be very put off or dismissive of the idea that he try yoga to deal with his problem. The power in gender roles is seen in the limits they put on action (i.e. how they might be used to shame someone) and in the penchant for universalizing in the person who has identified with them. We know that the misogynist and racist are saying more about themselves, when they claim that some personality traits are universal in women or minorities, than about those who they "other." Something very similar is happening with Gilbert and Gubar, and I will return to this idea later.

In *Transcending Gender* (1988), Joanne Blum's focus in on the *authentic intersubjectivity* that can be found between male and female characters. Blum wants to go beyond the traditional double who is a representation of "psychic fragmentation" and is projected into a hallucination or "shadow self" in a text (ibid., p. 3). Instead, the male/female pairs are viewed as "complete selves" that have an "interaction leading to a deeper awareness of selfhood and of relationship" (ibid., p. 3). She holds that because of patriarchal inequality, this meeting usually requires "extra-social placement." Blum includes sci-fi literature, for example, in which there is no physiological sex distinction between men and women as an example of such a space. However, in more traditional literature she holds that such a space can be seen in "spiritual bonds" that are registered outside of class or gender.

Blum does not use the psychoanalytic concept of psychic bisexuality, but refers to theorists who write of a *basic androgyny*. Although critical of this "bipolar construct" that is a "subtle reinforcement of gender polarity," she mentions a nascent development in the literature that is "less dichotomous," more "multidimensional," and "too complex for definition by gender" (ibid., p. 2). Blum also cites Nancy Chodorow's "asymmetrical relational experiences" in which mothers socialize girls differently to boys, to argue for a possible future reversibility of "feminine traits" (ibid., pp. 4–5). Despite this gesture towards a psychology with a dialectic between basic androgyny and gender roles, Blum exclusively focuses on the cultural conditioning of gender. The foundational claim is that gender identifications flow from the "tremendous degree to which society channels, categorizes, and restricts human behavior" (ibid., p. 10).

In her interpretation of *Jane Eyre* (1847), Blum begins by noting that the first meeting of Jane and Rochester is on the road when Jane assists him after he falls from his horse. This moment in their narrative is outside of the social world. Both characters recount the fairy tale-like nature of this encounter and establish the "mythic potential" of this space (Blum, 1988, p. 19). Despite this first encounter, Jane comes to work for Rochester and enters patriarchal space to find Rochester wants unearned respect or superiority. Jane continues to feel that outside of the rank and wealth that "severs" her from Rochester, that she is equal/similar to him on a mental plane (ibid., p. 20). Rochester also recognizes that Jane has an "inward treasure" that would grant Jane a satisfying life outside of any rank or authority in the social sphere. Blum holds that Rochester offers this recognition to Jane in a strange moment of the novel when he disguises himself as an old gypsy woman, and Jane, before she recognizes the ruse, feels a shared identity with the gypsy.

This equality on the mental level continues, but Jane is troubled by "unworthiness" on the social level. Rochester, on the latter level, attempts to mold Jane to be suitable to his station in life, but still manages to secure Jane's love on the mental level, until she discovers his wife, Bertha. Jane fears becoming a mere mistress, and Blum interprets Bertha as revealing a secret in Rochester's psyche: he perceives himself as a victim in the marriage, and does not see how he himself victimizes others. Blum believes this habit was "fostered by his social situation as privileged upper-class male" and is symbolic of Rochester's impediment to have equality with Jane in social space (ibid., p. 22). Although there is an important psychological statement here in regards to Rochester seeing himself as a victim, Blum again invokes gender roles and patriarchy as the culprit. He is not an agent with his own motivations for exploiting the laws or customs that favor his sex, but instead the social order itself "possesses" him and is the agent.

While Rochester symbolically works through his privilege, by having to deal with the fire that burns Bertha and his home, Blum holds that there is a parallel preparation that Jane must go through. She is tested through the figure of St. John who offers her marriage without the passionate love and equality Jane felt with Rochester. Blum again asserts the exclusivity of gender identity by writing that Jane's consideration of the marriage is from "the feminine code of passivity and self-sacrifice she has internalized" (ibid., p. 22). Interestingly, Blum does not note the contradiction between this and her former statements on Jane challenging Rochester's request for respect and superiority. Gender arises as a "deep interpretation" at every major moment of the text without textual support from the psychological descriptions of the characters. Again, it is possible that both men and women, after ego injuries, capitulate to the authority of gender norms and give up on desires outside of them, but this acquiescence has to be contrasted to visible psychological motivations.

Jane's bond to Rochester re-emerges in a telepathic, fantastical moment in the plot to provide an escape from St. John. Moreover, Jane inherits money from her uncle and becomes independent and now has the chance to have equality with Rochester on the social level. Blum interprets the injuries that Rochester received from the destruction of his home as a progressive moment that makes him learn to "lean on" or depend on Jane, and be aware of his responsibility for the events in his life (ibid., p. 23). Strangely, Blum is silent about Jane's proclamation to Rochester: "I love you better now, when I can be really useful to you." Jane was supposed to become St. John's "helpmate," and Blum ignores how this relation was carried over to Rochester. The focus remains on how their talk to each other is "but a more animated and an audible thinking," and the altruistic, Antigone-like role of Jane in the relationship, and the egoistic triumph of Jane's physical body over Rochester's, is ignored.

Instead of some biological essentialism that creates feminine psychology, we are given a discursive essentialism that is based on the socially constructed idea of "Woman." This is a strange incoherence in feminist theory. While feminists can recognize that attributing positive or negative traits to a minority is an untrue universalization, somehow a gender role is taken to have a universal impact upon women.[2] For example, to say that women are socialized to be competitive about their beauty and taste, is open to counterfactuals. We can recognize that not all women read beauty magazines or show this kind of competiveness with other women. Additionally, some men are competitive about their handsomeness or their superior taste too. However, perhaps Blum, like Gilbert and Gubar above, would say that there are many limiting gender roles that women can take on. Instead of being limited by "Womanness" in general, perhaps mothers "socialize" one sister to be more competitive about her looks and another is expected to be a Cinderella-figure who helps the mother out. There are certainly patients who have reported episodes from their past along such lines. The problem is what to make of situations in which sisters, for example, receive the same messages, and the parents valorize the same behaviors or traits for both siblings. When sisters turn out completely different in such cases, how can this difference be explained?[3] I know many progressive parents who have gone out of their way to give their sons dolls, pink clothing, etc., and not limit their daughters from activities associated with boys, and they can admit that they saw sexual differences emerge for which they do not feel responsible. Feminist thought is forced to double down here and claim that narratives and roles are subconsciously controlling the non-verbal behavior of even the feminists who strive to be neutral.[4] Claiming that the discourses of "Woman" subconsciously direct the motivations and desires of women, without them knowing it, is an interesting appropriation of the unconscious of psychoanalysis. However, it lacks the material basis upon which psychoanalysis founded its unconscious and, as it is used by Blum, it appears completely unfalsifiable.

It may be helpful to look at another type of example from individual psychology in order to appreciate the difference between the *first nature* of individual psychology and the *second nature* that culture can instill. For example, consider that a person, from psychosexual development, may have a schizoid economy of libido that makes him have a greater connection to the contents of his internal world than to the external world. For example, Frances Tustin (1988a, 1988b) powerfully describes amodal sensations that are sub-qualitative, and allow for autistic fixations that defend against connection with others. Such a first nature, for an individual on the spectrum, may allow an individual to be very stoic in relation to the loss of people and things in his life, and very introverted. There is a significant difference between someone who has this autistic fixation and who naturally could sit silently lost in sensations or contemplation and a person who learned to do this and exhibits it as second nature. For example, a child given to a monastery by a poor family, who does not have this fixation, can be forced to sit still, be punished for disobedience, and learn to overcome his first nature. He might have been inclined towards action and not any intellectualism or stoicism, but he can be forced to get in touch with this primitive stage of the mind. However, in contrast to the person on the autistic spectrum, he will be less in touch with the sense of pleasure and freedom of the activity and more dependent on the mantras, forms, and identifications with his teachers. I would like to suggest here that there are periods of history, and specific classes in them, in which second nature is not instilled or inscribed in people (or to a very diminished degree). Instead of acknowledging the reduction in second-nature inscription in our culture, we have increasing accounts of narratives that subconsciously and covertly inscribe it. If one makes room for individual psychology, then gender roles in the abstract are not as important as the dynamics of group psychology that use shame or bullying to cause the ego identifications.[5]

In line with explaining behavior through gender roles, Blum (1988) offers women the simple imperative of "recognizing and appreciating . . . the necessity of avoiding the trap of self-sacrifice and including self in the network of responsibilities" (p. 8). This kind of view fails on two accounts. First, for certain passive psychological types, for example, there is a desire to feel fostered by parental-substitutes. A mentor or stronger person's approval is required to feel comfortable with using one's skills or knowledge and one is open to an ego injury if one doesn't feel supported by them. However, there are men who have this problem too. *The Hobbit* film trilogy (2012–2014), for example, shows this relation between the protagonist Bilbo Baggins and the dwarf leader Thorin Oakenshield. The latter continually tells the former he is not a warrior and is too small and weak to be part of the quest. The dramatic tension in the film involves the former almost giving up due to this lack of fostering. I have had both male and female patients who register the desire to be fostered by a parental-substitute, who have the inability to say no, who get used by "friends," or who do for others while neglecting themselves. To say that this need for approval or issues with self-effacement are due to the internalization of feminine gender roles does not adequately explain this pattern in men.

The second issue concerns the efficacy of Blum's intellectual imperative to recognize the characterological problems of people pleasing, saying no, and self-effacement. These are traditionally considered issues of masochism in psychoanalysis—although I argue in *The Economics of Libido* (2015) that the term echoism is a more logical pairing with narcissism and has less ideological baggage. Echoists (masochists) can recognize that these things are an issue for them, but it does not assuage their fear that others might think they are mean or selfish if they begin to say no or put up boundaries. In my clinical experience these issues arise from projective identification with a good parental imago.[6] Citing gender roles that "have been psychologically internalized to [women's] detriment," is a very naïve way to talk about these issues, considering how there are people who leave the ivory tower to actually work with these issues in the clinic (Blum, 1988, p. 8). I would like to give a clinical vignette to illustrate the psychodynamics and imago relations in people with echoistic or "people-pleasing" traits:

Client begins the session by reporting that she's backed away from her older brother and as she details this, she begins to express that it has been to protect herself. She reports that he is always asking her for help and he is never there when she needs him for something. I ask for more details and she admits that she has a hard time saying no to him. I continue to press for an example and she says that she had given him $20 to fill up his car when she had no money, needed gas herself, and had actually ran out of gas afterwards. She has kids and is able to articulate why she shouldn't give him money when it's just going to make them suffer.

I ask client to picture her brother from the time she gave him the $20 and to tell him all the good reasons why she can't give him the $20, nor continue to help him as she has. I ask her to see what kind of response she imagines that he will give her in her mind's eye and begin BLS. After, she says that he looked "pessimistic," that he didn't accept her answer, that he said things to her like, "I'm going to lose my job" and "I can't do what I need to do," and was angry. She reports that she felt like backing down. I ask her if he is right and whether he is more important than her family, and she says no. She agrees to go back in to her mind's eye and try again.

After BLS client reports that he still doesn't accept what she says. I ask her to put into words what he's thinking about her. She says that he would be thinking things like "you owe this to me, I'd help you if you needed it, you're not worth talking to, you're selfish." I ask her to put these into ego and object statements about someone else (i.e. to think about who comes to mind when she thinks about someone the way her brother was thinking about her). She says a friend comes to mind. Client talks about this friend and how she wants to "guilt her" into listening to her problems, but one of her problems involves one of client's kids and client is angry about it. Although client knows her friend is in pain and wants to be there for her, client also feels like her friend is disregarding her feelings about her kid. As she talks, client begins to have an angry tone, I point this out to her and ask her where she feels it in her body and she reports that she feels tensions in her chest. I begin BLS in order to build up the feelings and then ask her when she has felt like this before. She says with her "mom" and I ask her for the first time that comes to mind with these feelings.

She says that her mom should have been more "protective" and that she "placed [client] in harm's way" when she left her with a relative. Client says her dad "worked a lot," wasn't there either, and describes how bad it could get with this relative. Client mentions how she told her mother about what happened later in life and that her mother was dismissive and was neither compassionate nor took accountability. I tell client that no child should have had to deal with what she had to go through and ask how her mother could be so unsympathetic. Client continues on this line and expresses frustration that she has had to feel like her emotions make her a burden and adds in exasperation that she "didn't ask to be born." As she continues to build anger over this, I tell her to go back into this memory and this time, to picture her mother and tell her what she's told me. I begin BLS and tell her to put everything into words until she feels the anger and tension in her chest have been expressed. I add that she should then tell me what her mother looks like and how she reacts. After BLS, client says that she feels like she "got rid of her anger" but that her mother looked "cold." "She knows I'm right," client begins, "but to admit that I'm right is too much for her." After a moment of silence, she adds that her mother "can't handle being wrong" and that "she has to be perfect."

I get client to continue talking about how her mother cares what she looks like to others, but doesn't care about what she actually does, or how she actually treats her children. Client shows strong insight into how her mother would get defensive and she brings up other situations in which she couldn't be wrong. I ask her if she has ever told her mother about how she can see through her and she says no. I explain to her that parents have to pass on their "adultness" to their children, so that the children can feel confident about being adults and not like kids who feel like they are frauds or just pretending to be grown up. I point out that her mother never gave this to her, but if she doesn't tell her mother that she can see through her, then she will let her mother keep this and will never feel "adult" herself. Client agrees and I tell her to say this to her "cold, perfect" mother and speak her truth, and begin BLS. Client looks much softer and calmer when she signals for me to stop, and tells me that afterwards her mother looked "almost broken" and "human." I ask her to focus on the way her mother now looks in her mind's eye and to pay attention to how her body reacts to this picture and resume BLS. Client reports feeling strong "relief" from the feeling that "something might actually be there," behind her mother's perfect image. Client takes several more breaths and says "my mom never got to be an adult either," and talks about what she knows about her mother and her childhood. After this, I ask client to go back into the memory with her brother and to now tell him again that she needs the money for herself and her family. I begin BLS and tell her to tell me what he looks like when the scene plays out. After, she tells me that he had "apologized" and that she had said, "everything I lack on my end comes back down on me, my family, I could lose the house." She reports that he had said, "you're right, and I'm sorry." She feels like she can tell him no and he won't get mad and want to stay away from her, and reports as much in the following session.

My patient had been in PI with the good parental imago, which is part of the passive pole of the personality. By taking the description of what her brother would think of her if she said no, and asking her to consider how she has felt like him with people in her life, this defensive position was reversed. She had not felt protected by her mother and, in PI, she took over the place of the good parent that she had needed her mother to be, while her brother played out the neediness that she defended against. Despite this defense, she appeared to partially put her friend in the position of parental-substitute and expressed this frustration, as a link to the original ego injury with her mother. After showing courage by confronting her mother in her mind's eye, she was able to repair the injury and show assertiveness with her brother in both fantasy and then in real life. I have seen behavioral interventions work when patients have enough transference to their therapist to be motivated to act in a new and very uncomfortable way. However, the idea that simply having male parents do more of the caregiving, or offering slogans for the empowerment of women is a very superficial view of the psychology involved in this.

Social constructivism also leads Blum's account into other troubling waters. She notes that the solitary life that Jane and Rochester lead is barely a part of the social sphere except for some annual visits from family. This state of affairs is interpreted as an example of how a relationship of equality in the gender-transcendent bond is antithetical to the world's patriarchy. So interpreted, this resembles Fredric Jameson's claim that "it is easier to imagine the end of the world than to imagine the end of capitalism" (Jameson, 2003, p. 73). Disaster movies that show asteroids threatening the earth, for example, are supposed to show a failure to imagine a new social organization. For Blum, the parallel would be that it is easier to imagine telepathic communication, or fantastic worlds in which no sexual difference exists, than it is to imagine a genuine relationship of equality in our patriarchal culture. Gilbert and Gubar's idea that female artists should be creating new gender roles could be added here as well. The question is whether artists or novelists who create new worlds or characters, or depict the destruction of their world or one of their characters, should be understood to be doing so, based upon some normative, progressively political sense?

Teleological considerations of what a totally authentic and fair future social organization, or new form of gender identity may look like, are, at best, indulgence in a philosophical position of dialectical idealism. The position of the dialectical idealist is that ideas and narratives are what have power and make changes in the social order. For example, the idealist may look at the past with the view that if a president like Abraham Lincoln would have ascended into power sooner, then slavery would also have ended sooner in America. This kind of idealist vision is assumed without an appreciation of the technological advancements and group psychology necessary to effect such changes. Such a view is held, in echoistic denial, of the powerful racism that existed at that time. Moreover, when a classic leftist would be reminded of the racism at that time, often his position would be that "deep down, people are good" and this racism could be overcome with simple education. This ideological view fails to appreciate how the racists of that time would hardly swallow their pathological pride and simply join Blacks, side by side, to work on the plantation. Additionally, it conveys a naïve sense of the psychological defenses at play in racism. In contrast, the Marxian view is that with increased industrialization in the North, and the changes this brought to labor practices and social life, racism was modified in a new social organization that was forced upon the South. The latter development would reference the economic interest of the elites who controlled the new technology and factories in the North, although this kind of change is represented in the public eye as the triumph of ideals and altruism.

Marx's great insight is that egoism is the motor of history. The self-interest of a lower class, once it is paired with technological advancements, causes them to overthrow the elite with the by-product of an increase of rights. In other words, the new masters rally the people against the old masters, so that they can be in charge, while representing it to the people as an issue of rights and liberty. Altruistic concern alone is not enough to stand up against the weight of tradition and the transference to authority.

In another example, women's rights and their emergence into the work and political world, did not arise from men finally being persuaded by arguments for the equality of women. Instead, male opposition to women's rights was broken down by things like male capitalists employing women because they could pay them less money, or capitalists putting them in factories during a war because of necessity. When people grew accustomed to seeing and hearing about women in these roles, and the "seal was broken," more of the population tolerated this change. The egoism of the capitalists ate away at the strong traditions of keeping women in the home, before it paired with the altruistic concern for women's rights in the public eye.

It is the valorization of "naked self-interest" in capitalism, which issued from the technological infrastructure of the previous political economy, which allowed women new freedoms. Social life was such that the narcissists who did not care about bad reputations in the community were allowed to flout such traditions, without the community forcing them to toe the line. This is what distinguishes capitalism from previous political economies in which money existed (ex. Ancient Greece). However, to be a dialectical materialist also means that one recognizes that there is some work done at the level of discourse and narratives as well. For example, Marx in *On the Jewish Question* (1844a) credits Christianity with "sever[ing] all the species-ties of man." These species-ties previously allowed the community to use religion, or other forms of group solidarity, to check or inhibit individuals in the community who were being too greedy in their accumulation. Presumably, Marx is indicating something like the idea that Christianity increased self-absorption and preoccupation with one's own soul (ex. making it to heaven) to the detriment of good works in the community. Then, while the spiritual types of people who could have a strong effect on the group psychology of the community were so preoccupied, an increase of consumerism and other material practices would enter into society in order to preserve this change.[7]

It is doubtful that Hegel was actually a dialectical idealist in the way discussed above, but it is clear that Marx is at least critical of how the philosophy of Hegel was received by the dialectical idealists who followed him. He writes:

> Since the Young Hegelians consider conceptions, thoughts, ideas, in fact all the products of consciousness, to which they attribute an independent existence, as the real chains of men (just as the Old Hegelians declared them the true bonds of human society) it is evident that the Young Hegelians have to fight only against these illusions of consciousness. Since, according to their fantasy, the relationships of men, all their doings, their chains and their limitations are products of their consciousness, the Young Hegelians logically put to men the moral postulate of exchanging their present consciousness for human, critical or egoistic consciousness, and thus of removing their limitations. This demand to change consciousness amounts to a demand to interpret reality in another way, i.e. to recognise it by means of another interpretation. The Young-Hegelian ideologists, in spite of their allegedly "world-shattering" statements, are the staunchest conservatives. The most recent of them have found the correct expression for their activity when they declare they are only fighting against "phrases." They forget, however, that to these phrases they themselves are only opposing other phrases, and that they are in no way combating the real existing world when they are merely combating the phrases of this world.
>
> *(Marx, 1845a)*

The idealist position in Gilbert and Gubar, Jameson, and Blum is to assume that we must fly ahead in thought. In their cases, the idealist imagines that artists and thinkers should be anticipating some new, perfect (or closer to perfect) future. The unuttered assumption here is that future changes in culture will arise *ex nihilo*: new gender roles and new social arrangements will arise from some understanding of the insidious ways that men and women are controlled. This idealist stance is in stark contrast to Marx's dialectical materialism in which technology, economics, and ideational content silently change how people interact. Marx does not give a detailed plan of what communism will look like—as if society will be made to resemble a dogmatic conception of how some think we should be living ethically. Communism is something he can point to because he was the first thinker to direct our attention to the changes of class interactions in the past.[8]

Instead of seeing the artist as creating out of a failure to see through ideology, I would argue that the failure is with the theorist who wants to look away from concrete praxis and real social life. At some future point, thinkers will see how social relations have qualitatively changed and then, along with psychologists, they will interpret a new *superstructure*. On one hand, these ideas will show how the capitalist system is a limitation on both the productive forces in society and, on the other, they will concern new visions of group identity that go beyond the old, alienating influences of religious mysticism, racism, misogyny, etc. The key is that the new social organization cannot be a new social contract in which the religious, for example, simply agree to stop worshipping. Instead, psychologists will have to prove themselves in praxis and show that they can help people to enjoy enough satisfaction in this world, that they choose to let go of their belief in the next one. The new social organization will not begin by the majority of people accepting and wanting to submit to the intellectual and moral elitism of the students of the humanities.

The third school of double scholarship is an idealism that reifies gender roles and leaves behind any clinical grounding in depth structures. Although the critics I examined do not represent it in this way, their interpretations of the characters, or their authors, effectively makes them doubles of the patriarchal social order. The symptom reading that I will begin to introduce in the next chapter should be understood as issuing from the second school of double scholarship.

Instead of just constructing an emotional insight into a character through his or her double, a whole latent plot will be created. This latent plot will also provide a limit to manic doubling, which offers no insight into a character's relationship or reaction to an event. However, the symptom reading also draws part of its impetus in opposing the third school's insistence on cultural conditioning by providing a more comprehensive psychoanalytic theory of personality. Through providing a close reading of *The Lost Boys* (1987) I will show how a five-step procedure suggested itself in multiple viewings of the film and re-readings of the script.

Notes

1 In Chapter 5, when I introduce the deutero phase and the phallic mother, it will be possible to see how characters like Rochester can be interpreted as frustrating parental-substitutes. This also makes sense of idiosyncrasies in the story, such as when Rochester dresses up like an old gypsy woman, because the phallic mother relation is transcribed to the paternal in some relations, but still can carry its original feminine images. Darth Vader in the original *Star Wars* trilogy has feminine elements in his helmet shape and cloak, and is another example of this.

2 Similarly, some cultural theorists will try to claim that there is an "American" subject, or some Americanness that informs every citizen's identity. However, when we see how polarized things can be between Republican and Democrat, and how politicians in both parties try to pander and appeal to people in very different ways, it is difficult to see how traits of "Americanness" can really be shared across these two major political groupings in any deep way. As mentioned above, what is American is a cultural ideal that is more notable for what it prohibits/how it's used to shame (i.e. "It's un-American to do X") and in the specific individuals who self-consciously want to hang American flags, eat American foods, shop American, etc.

3 A similar encounter with psychology is found in the fact that gay or lesbian parents (i.e. two fathers or two mothers) don't produce gay or lesbian children in a statistically significant increase that would, for example, reverse the 1 in 10 homosexual children (from straight parents) to 9 out of 10.

4 The open-mindedness of parents who don't feel like they have an agenda for their children, should be contrasted to parents who can consciously say that they did not know how to raise a girl so they treated their daughter like a boy, for example. Similarly, patients have also told me how their son reminded them of his abusive father and so they avoided things that might make him angry, or they had no friends and so they got their son to comb their hair and put make up on him, like he was a childhood girlfriend.

5 Similarly, American exceptionalism and the conservative traditions of some states should not be viewed as a totally contingent identity. Rather, narcissistic individuals who chose to leave their (extended) family and community in order to chase superlative success, surely impact the group psychology in their new homes. Ego identifications with them,

and their motivational structures, is part of the confluence of forces that make a given group identity salient.

6 The good parental imago is a reference to the parental imago who would foster the individual and give approval and/or protection. It will be examined more with the passive pole of psychic bisexuality beginning in the next book.

7 Marx's insight is to see that "human essence is no abstraction inherent in each single individual," from the "internal, dumb generality" of social discourse (Marx, 1845b, sec. 6). In discussing worldviews like Christianity, Marx argues that they are formed from "an ensemble of the social relations," which is different from his views of religion as a tool of the political elite and the opiate of the masses (ibid.) Marx doesn't offer any catalogue or taxonomy of psychological types, but in his early work, he highlights that he perceives and recognizes deep differences between individuals: "Assume *man* to be *man* and his relationship to the world to be a human one: then you can exchange love only for love, trust for trust, etc. . . . if you want to exercise influence over other people, you must be a person with a stimulating and encouraging effect on other people. Every one of your relations to man and to nature must be a *specific expression* . . . of your *real individual* life. If you love without evoking love in return—that is, if your loving as loving does not produce reciprocal love; if through a *living expression* of yourself as a loving person you do not make yourself a *beloved one*, then your love is impotent—a misfortune" (Marx, 1844b). Marx does not claim that communism will make everyone capable of loving or in possession of charisma. Instead, part of his concept of alienation includes how work in capitalism can often ignore these "ontological affirmations of essential being" (ibid.). Instead of taking a management role because one is a natural leader, for example, someone can take on this role because of inheritance or nepotism, or because he promises stockholders to raise profits through the further mechanization of job duties, or firing employees before they get retirement benefits.

8 Marx obviously made an error in assuming that Communism would arise during his lifetime and that there was not more work for capitalism to do in regards to reducing the importance of religion, racism, and other worldviews of the past. However, his hope for something to occur in his day does not invalidate his approach to studying social change, nor does it make his thought responsible for the bastardizations of twentieth-century socialism.

4

THE SYMPTOM READING (PART 1)

"My blood is in your veins"

Since I am introducing a new methodology, I thought it would be important to share my thought process after encountering the narrative in *The Lost Boys* (1987). Watching this film, I was first struck by the loosely oedipal triangle that takes place in the triangle of David, Star, and Michael. I say loosely oedipal because Michael sees a mysterious, beautiful girl, Star, who seems interested in him too, but she is somehow attached to another man, David. She's not David's girlfriend or, at least, he is not portrayed as having a romantic interest in her. David is the leader of the lost boys and has a superior motorcycle, representative of his superiority to Michael. In the script notes for the film, the comparison between the two bikes is made explicit, and Michael is described as "out-classed" by David's "throbbing" motorcycle. Although Michael and David appear to be equally matched in strength, or force of will, at the end of the film—with Michael defeating him—David is represented as at least having an advantage over Michael in earlier scenes. I would also argue that in some of them David seems much more powerful and toys with Michael. In one such scene, David causes Michael to hallucinate maggots and worms; in another, he challenges Michael to a race and the latter almost rides off a cliff.

Despite Star's apparent connection to David, David seems more focused on getting Michael to enter his group of lost boys than he is in competing with him for Star's affection. Even up to the last battle, when all of the other lost boys have been killed by Michael and his group, David still wants Michael to become a full vampire and "join him." Through multiple dialogues between the two characters in the film, it becomes clear that David's interest in Michael is practically obsessive.

Michael possesses no special characteristics of circumstances that warrant David's excessive interest in him. He is not given a back story of special intelligence, strength, ties to the occult, etc., and does not appear to have any special merit except his teen-age appeal as an attractive, brooding loner. At the end of the story, Max emerges as the head vampire, and we find out that David's special interest in Michael stems from Max's interest in marrying Lucy so she can help him better control his "lost boys." However, the idea of making her into the "bride of Dracula," as if she will have special power to "mother" David and the others, or get them to listen to what Max wants them to do, seems strange. *The Lost Boys* is largely a fantastical horror story, and therefore questions about what is "realistic" might seem out of place, but who is Lucy to them? If she is supposed to have some special virtue of kindness that they will respect, how could she respect herself for being complicit in the murders they commit as they feed off of humans? In the script, Max's intended role for Lucy is different, she is supposed to become the "daytime guardian" for the vampires. But, how would an older woman protect them? Max is rich, what would prevent him from hiring a strong bodyguard and saying he is a relative? Moreover, if Max wants to live anonymously in the suburbs, what will people think as Lucy ages and Max and "their boys" never age? This plot point was troubling for me and in the second part of the reading I put together an answer for it in the latent plot that is a much more plausible motivation.

If we bracket the troubling point of Max instructing David to get Michael to join him, there are essentially two parallel plots up to this point. David is portrayed as the leader of the lost boys for most of the story and Max is only revealed to be the true leader at the end. Max's coming out as head vampire gives a rationalization as to why David was so interested in Michael, but what if David's interest is just taken at face value? Michael's relationship with Star and David and Sam's relationship with Lucy and Max cross over at some points, but the former involves fantastical figures, while the latter is more reality-based.[1] These triangles function as parallels—the way David feels about Michael shows how Max feels about Sam. David's reference to how "[his] blood is in [Michael's] veins" is easy enough to relate to family "blood relations." Max does not have the same blood as Sam, but if he marries his mother, Max still becomes "man of the house" and can put rules and discipline in place. Sam could come to regard him as a father figure. My analysis will show that there is textual evidence that Max has a special interest in how Sam should be raised, which suggests he wants to take on a formative or parental role in Sam's life, and that David's desire to enlist Michael is the overt expression of this.

The interactions between Michael and David are just one part of their triangle, the other part is the relation between Michael and Star. Michael has a romantic interest in Star, and there is a scene in which Sam spends the night in Lucy's bed because he is "scared" that his brother might be a vampire. I do not mean to imply that Sam commits incest with his mother, but only that there could be loving or affectionate feelings that are part of his motivations here. Again, even though the two plots overlap at times, they remain separate; it is not until the twist ending that the fantastical elements are confirmed for Max and Lucy in Sam's plot. Before this, Sam's triangle largely involves events around his mom dating her boss—a more familiar, realistic, domestic plot. Rather than consider these two plots in isolation, however, I suggest an interpretation of the film wherein this domestic plot is the central psychological drama of the film, and the vampire plot functions as a space of fantasy and as the unconscious symptom for Sam's triangle.

Reading the film in this way puts its neurotic glory on full display. A boy moves with his mother to live with her father after her divorce and every time his mother goes on a date with her boss, he makes up a crazy story to sabotage those dates. Every time Sam sabotages the dates between Max and Lucy he references his brother being a vampire or the threat of vampires in general. By invoking the fantastical elements related to Michael's plot, then the desires and fears of the Michael–Star–David triangle are expressed in the Sam–Lucy–Max triangle. Sam's reference to them in his plot is the rationalization of how they are expressed in his plot.

The symptom reading is so named because this dialectical formulation resembles what Freud (1900) divined in his concept of a symptom (pp. 569–570). A symptom both allows the expression of an unconscious desire and, at the same time, only reveals this desire in hidden form. In one of Freud's examples, a woman has hysterical vomiting in which the wish to have children is expressed by the association of the vomiting to the morning sickness of pregnancy but, manifestly, this desire is masked in the conscious mind. A symptom is also an expression of the need for punishment, in which castration anxiety is avoided by the impulses that are tied to anxiety-producing interactions being turned against the self. "Castration" in psychoanalysis is a general way of referring to anxiety situations at different psychosexual stages (i.e. phallic, anal, etc.) that may concern the loss or damage to genitalia but also fear of disapproval from authority figures, fear for life (i.e. death), fear of abandonment, etc. (Freud, 1926a). In Freud's example, the hysterical morning sickness also threatens his patient with the loss of her good looks and figure. This aspect is very important and concerns the *economics of punishment* and *apathy* that I will define and discuss in the next book.

As mentioned above, when Michael meets Star he sees that she has some non-romantic tie to David and his group of lost boys. Later we learn that she is a half vampire and has some of David's blood in her too. This can be interpreted as Sam feeling like his mother has a special tie to, or properly belongs to, an adult male (i.e. she wouldn't be romantically interested in boys, let alone her own son). Just as Michael tries to steal Star away from David, we can interpret Sam as trying to steal Lucy away from Max as her appropriately aged partner. Additionally, despite this relation of Sam stealing Lucy from Max, there is a sense in which Sam possesses her. For example, Max tells Sam that he *is not* trying to "replace his dad or steal his mom," and implies that she belongs to Sam in some way. Again, this is not solely about Sam having his mother's love, but also involves, as dialogue in the film suggests, who will be "man of the house." To the extent that David's relation in the triangle can be transcribed to Max, then Michael's resistance to becoming a vampire, and joining David's group is how Sam would feel about Max being head of the family. Michael does not want to become a murderer like David, and Sam can be interpreted as having some sense that this new adult male is "bad" and, as his protégé, he would become bad too. Again, Max coming out as head of the vampires at the end will complicate this analysis, but the excision of Michael's character and plot, and the dialectical step of Michael both expressing and rationalizing the desires and fears of the triangle, is the beginning of the data analysis.

Data analysis I

David and Max are both linked by being "head vampire" and being in the position of leader of a group/family. Star is connected to David through his vampire blood, and Lucy is connected to Max as her age-appropriate partner, and Michael shares identity with Sam through being his brother. In Michael's triangle with Star and David, we get to watch Michael meet and fall in love with Star. Even though Michael sees that Star is part of David's gang, and that she rides on his motorbike, he tries to get time with her, win her affection, and this culminates in him breaking into the crypt of the vampires to steal her away. On the other side of the triangle, the side emphasizing power and authority, David's strange insistence that Michael join him and his lost boys, is the central relation. Despite the fact that Michael, Sam, and the Frog brothers stole Star away, destroyed one of the lost boys in their abandoned hotel lair, and then destroyed the rest of David's group at the final showdown, David still wants Michael. In this relation, David sees Michael's independence and wants him under his authority, but Michael wants to be his "own man" and struggles to resist becoming a killer and immoral like the vampires.

The symptomatic or dialectical aspect of the reading began for me with the principle of excising Michael's plot and looking for the moments that Michael, or the fantastical elements of his plot, were mentioned, or had an effect on Sam's plot. For example, when Lucy is on her first date with Max, Lucy calls to check up on Sam. He tells his mother that they have to have a "long talk" about something and when he sees his brother, Michael, floating outside of his window he exclaims, "Oh, no! Oh, God! He's coming to get me! Mom!!!" Lucy instantly runs out of her date to get to her son. Michael convinces Sam that he should not tell their mother he is a (half-) vampire and so Sam "lies" when she gets home, telling Lucy that he made a mistake and hallucinated a vision outside of the window. Sam tells her that he got "a little carried away" while reading a horror comic and the script expresses how Lucy regards this "with a good deal of skepticism."

At this point in the timeline, the narrative plays with the tension between the suspension of disbelief about the supernatural and the sense that we are being presented with the skewed perception of one of the characters. The viewer is unsure if she will soon come to see that the supernatural event (Michael floating by the window) really occurred or not. Earlier in the film David had "tricked" Michael into seeing the Chinese food he offered him as worms and maggots instead of noodles and rice, and then reverted them back again. The "reality" of perceptions in the film and the true form (the foul faces) of the vampires are not yet confirmed. Lucy's skepticism, as the parent, also influences the viewer. The realistic way in which she sees Sam here, and at later parts of the film is an important guide for building the latent plot.

With the excision of Michael's plot, we should actually take Sam's "lie," about getting ideas about vampires from reading comic books, as the case. However, instead of taking him to be an innocent, naïve boy whose imagination carries him away, we should look to the relation between Michael, Star, and David as the motivation. Sam lies not to protect Michael, but as an expression of his desire to possess his mother and steal her from Max as well as to remain his "own man." His lie is an expression of the desire for both affection and love from her, and to remain the "man of the house" as Max calls Michael. When Sam tells his mother that they need to have a "long talk," its meaning, with the excision of Michael's plot, points to his unhappiness with Lucy's date.

Along with the symptom reading explanation of Sam's motivations, there are *script slip* links between the symptom and ego characters. Two important such slips are shown after Sam ruins his mother's date, later that night, when he asks to sleep in bed with her, citing the "horror comic" he read. Again, the experience of Sam seeing that Michael is (becoming) a vampire, provides him a rationalization for sleeping in bed with his mother. Instead of a "long talk," Sam probably hopes that being close to her might help keep things the same or soothe his anxiety about losing her. The first script slip here, or link between ego and symptom characters, occurs after Sam gets into bed with his mother. The shot soon goes to Sam and Lucy sleeping and then the viewer sees Sam's eyes blinking open after he hears a motorbike driving off. The viewer's last memory of a motorbike is David playing a game of chicken with Michael that almost resulted in Michael riding over a cliff to his death. The motorbike sound in this scene links the signal anxiety (death/castration) that Michael experienced in his rivalry with David, to the relationship of how Sam feels about Lucy when he's lying in bed with her. The parallel in the structure of anxiety is that David is represented as superior or more "adult" than Michael and his competition with David is a rivalry with a parental-substitute. In Sam's case, it is easy to call out the transgression of the incest taboo in Sam getting into bed with his mother, whether it concerns love/affection or registers how Lucy is closer to him than to Max.[2]

The second script slip is that the song playing when Sam is in bed with his mother continues to play as the ego plot switches to the symptom plot. The motorbike revving turns out to be coming from Michael, who rides to the home of the lost boys to find Star. When he arrives there, he locates Star's bed and falls asleep there, only to be woken by voices and Star herself coming to lie down with him. He tells her that he has to talk to her, but rather than respond, she falls into a deep sleep from which he cannot wake her. Finally, as if still asleep, she murmurs to him to meet her that night at the boardwalk, at which point the exegetic music ceases. The song gives continuity between the two scenes beyond their adjacency in the narrative of the film. I take this replication of Star and Michael being in bed, with Star sleeping and Michael awake, right after we are given the scene of Lucy and Sam in bed, with Lucy sleeping and Sam awake, as a powerful link. Moreover, Michael's request to talk to Star is an echo of Sam saying "Mom. I think we've got to have a long talk about something" before his fear of Michael causes him to cry out.

This adjacent scene with the tie of music and parallels between the two pairs is just one of several links between the two pairs of "lovers." Early in the film, the shots of Michael being mesmerized and following Star are cut with shots of Lucy: their adjacent relation sets up their equivalence as the image of Star *becomes* the image of Lucy. Additionally, in an early scene we can see the equivalence expressed in language, when Sam interrupts an exchange between Star and Michael on the boardwalk with the announcement that "mom's here." By declaring "mom's here," Sam is both announcing that his mother is on the boardwalk and, following the imagistic linking of Star and Lucy, he saying Star *is* mom. I really must stress that after doing the symptom reading a few times it is surprising how apparent the narrative links between the symptom and ego character in images really is.

The next important script slip is when Lucy takes Sam with her to Max's house to drop off a bottle of wine as a gift, and apology, for running out of their date. It should be recalled that Michael became a "half-vampire" after he was tricked into drinking David's blood in a wine bottle. This links the important relation of paternity to more than just the phallic shape of the bottle. By Lucy bringing a bottle of wine to Max, the link between David initiating his blood claim to paternity over Michael and Lucy giving similar power to Max with her gift is established. This comes into greater relief in the next scene.

Max's next date with Lucy is at her father's house, where she and Sam are living. Here the rivalry between David and Michael finds explicit expression in the relation between Max and Sam. First, Max and Lucy's date is again disrupted when Sam invites himself and his friends, the Frog brothers, to dinner. Sam and his friends believe that Max might be a vampire because he only works at night and his dog nearly attacked Lucy when she had brought over the bottle of wine during the day. Again, with the excision of the symptom characters, the rationalizing of Sam testing Max to see if he's a vampire is only a pretense for Sam to covertly express Michael's relation to his triangle. Sam introduces himself just as Max is about to kiss Lucy in the kitchen. The next aggressive maneuver takes place when Sam offers Max cheese for his spaghetti at the dinner table. The cheese is actually garlic and the quantity of it causes him to choke. Another such aggressive moment occurs when Sam offers Max water to help clear his throat, but then intentionally spills it on his lap. Holy water is supposed to burn a vampire (Sam explicitly asks Max afterwards if it burns), and the thus it is something of a castration attempt. Finally, the Frog brothers turn off the lights and hold up a mirror before Max since, in classical lore, vampires cannot see their reflections in mirrors. Max passes this test as well, and ends the evening with a speech to the boys and Lucy, expressing his thoughts about her being a single mother. Max tells Sam that he does not want to take the place of his father nor "steal" his mother, then tells Lucy boys like Sam need to have "discipline, or they walk all over you."

This implies that, despite his protestations about interloping, he is offering to fill the position of paternal authority figure, and does want to replace Sam's dad.[3] Additionally, this scene also establishes that Lucy feels a resistance to accepting Max as a paternal authority. There are directions that she reacts "defensively" to Max's remarks that she allows her boys to walk all over her in the script. This defensiveness is parallel to Star's attempt to resist her impulses to feed/kill and move from half- to full-vampire under David's authority. Although she agrees to a third date, this misgiving about Max, along with Sam's resistance to him, register as the Michael and Star parallel to David.

There is a great script slip when Max first showed up for the dinner, and makes an out-of-place remark about how diners should not see the food before dinner. Lucy corrects him that this is said about the groom should not see the bride, and Max responds by saying that he "always" confuses those two ideas. On one hand, this bad joke works with the tension of whether or not Max is the head vampire, as Sam and the Frog brothers believe him to be at this point, and thus could be read as foreshadowing Lucy as potential food. However, the comment also registers the intention for paternity since it shows that Max is not thinking just about dating Lucy, but marrying her. From the egocentric position of Sam, the primary ego character in the triangle, marriage would for surely mean that Max would lead the family and likely include providing Sam with the discipline he "needs."

Lastly, the script calls for a "shame-faced" reaction in Sam after Max declares that he does not want to replace his dad or steal his mom. For him to feel shame after the speech, as opposed to after Max had failed all the vampire tests, shows that the content of the speech *is* how Sam feels. In the symptom reading, in which only the ego characters or reality-based plot comprise the latent narrative, Max's reading of Sam's intentions is the shameful truth. Otherwise, if Sam felt shame for ruining the date and being aggressive towards an innocent man, we would expect him to apologize or try to set things right with Max, but no such actions follow this. Moreover, Max's speech is very empathic and kind. Although a kid might feel ashamed just at being "in trouble," the speech does not reprimand Sam in anyway. I want to stress again that Max, in guessing Sam's intentions, is giving a reality-based interpretation of what is happening, while the viewer is distracted by the symptom plot involving vampires. In the symptom reading, we are often only following the cues given by the reality-based viewpoint embedded in the narrative itself.

The next important part of the latent plot is when Max and Lucy are going to meet for their third attempt at a date. This date is preceded, and rationalized by, an important event in the symptom plot. Just as Sam and the Frog brothers attempted to attack Max (feed him garlic, holy water on the genitals), they join Michael to attack David and in order to steal Star away. Star had expressed that she wanted to be with Michael and did not want to be a vampire, but she had mysteriously vanished when she received some kind of telepathic communication or sensed that David was looking for her. Michael, Sam, and the Frog brothers steal Star and Laddie, a small boy who is also a half-vampire, knowing that David will seek his revenge for this and for them killing one of the lost boys. This state of affairs is the rationalization for Sam to try to break up Lucy and Max's re-scheduled third date, and is likely based on his expectation that Max will want revenge for how Sam and the Frog brothers treated him at dinner.[4]

Prior to their date, Sam attempts to alert his mother to the vampire presence in Santa Clara. Lucy sees this as a bid to foil another date with Max and tells Sam not to "ruin it" yet again, to which Sam responds, "to hell with Max!" Again, we are given the coordinates for making the symptom reading by the narrative itself. Lucy, like any reasonable person, does not believe in vampires; Sam's behavior, for her, can only be seen as a reaction to her romance with Max. Although, the viewer could well identify with Sam's "exploding" curse, "to hell with Max," given what is going on in the symptom plot, the same curse takes on another meaning with the excision off the symptom plot: "to hell with Max" is explosive anger at the realization that Lucy has guessed Sam's real intentions and hatred of his rival, Max.

In the last scene in the ego plot, before the final battle in the symptom plot, Max establishes himself as a real rival. Lucy reacted poorly to Max's previous approach of exclaiming the need for paternal authority—for him—in the family, by implying Sam walked all over Lucy. Here he changes his tactics in order to get her mind off of Sam's frantic request for her to inform the authorities about the vampires in the city (i.e. his dislike of Max). On the date, Max asks Lucy why she's distracted, and she responds that her mind is on her sons, "as usual." This conversation includes a reversal of Max's position, and now he tells Lucy that boys should be "ignored" and turn out best that way. Lucy brings up the reversal but Max cleverly self-depreciates that a bachelor like him cannot claim to know much on this subject and this culminates in their first real kiss.

This kiss between Max and Lucy is important because up to this point they had only had two failed dates. As I mentioned above, I think what is important here is that there is the sense that Lucy belongs with an adult sexual partner, not a child, but the kiss allows Max to register as the one who is in that structural position. The vampire blood and telepathy in the symptom plot are fantastic connections to represent an important structure in the mind (i.e. the difference between the generations in the Oedipus complex that I will introduce in the next chapter). As mentioned above, Star leaves Michael in one scene because David was looking for her and manifests a telepathic connection with her through their blood tie. Max's kiss with Lucy represents a similar connection that Sam knows he cannot have with his mother.

I have taken to calling the next part of symptom reading, *the navel* of the symptom. To be clear, the term is not used as Freud uses it for dream interpretation. For Freud (1900), it means the part of the dream that cannot be understood. For the symptom reading, it means the part of the action that happens in the symptom plot that is not shown in the ego plot. When Michael resists the call of David's blood (i.e. joining his "family" or group) and kills him, there is an implied parallel that Sam dispatches with his rival, Max. Perhaps, Lucy's worrying got the better of her and she tells Max that she has to go home and check on him. He offers to come with her, and they see that Sam had trashed the house out of anger. It is possible that Max decides that he does not want to deal with Sam and, in this way, he reveals himself in his immoral aspect (just as the vampires are indifferent to the feelings of those that they kill and feed upon). However, this interpretation is not satisfying and, moreover, does not follow the structure that a symptom character is paired with an ego character.

After David is killed, Max reveals himself as head vampire, and thus leaves the ego plot and enters the symptom plot. Max coming out in this way makes his speech resonate with the latent plot that has been constructed. He tells Lucy that this "was all going to be so perfect," with his lost boys and Lucy's boys together in "one big happy family." In excising the symptom plot, Max is showing that his interest, first and foremost, was in having a family with Lucy, and therefore being Sam's father. Again, following the logic of the text, it is bizarre that a vampire would want a middle-aged woman to be his guardian or to somehow give him control over the young men he has changed into vampires. How would Lucy stop any attackers? The vampires, with all their powers, could get as much money as they want and could hire bodyguards, ex-marines, etc. to protect them. How long could Lucy last before she's enfeebled by old age, if not driven mad by the killing her "family" does? Moreover, why does Max say he still wants her even after he enters and sees that his "sons" are all destroyed? Max's intentions in the symptom plot make little sense, but they might if we determine who Max's ego character is, after he becomes a symptom character. However, this data analysis should provide enough material for a basic overview of the psychoanalytic model of mind, clarify the triangles in the film, and lay the foundation for the second data analysis.

Notes

1 There are arguably more distinct plots since Sam and the Frog brothers have their own dynamic going on that can be separated from the other two plots. In the second half of the symptom reading I will turn to the Frog brothers and how the latent plot involves them and Grandpa too.

2 It is important to follow the structure of the text if the data analysis is to yield authentic data, and not just stretch readings to merely fit existing psychoanalytic concepts. In doing so, important distinctions in the psychoanalytic model of personality can be made and debates between different schools can be resolved.

3 Negations and disavowals actually meaning affirmation or avowal in psychoanalysis are an easy observation to criticize, but it is a valuable clinical tool when approached with subtlety. Not every negation is an avowal. Only those in which the quantity of disavowals is significant or the patient strangely discounts the possibility of something the analyst, and any "regular person," would not have been anticipating the disavowed aspect in the narrative the patient was weaving. For example, when a patient describes an unknown person in a dream and tells you that he or she doesn't think it's his or her father, when there was no reason to guess that it was, you can often take a description of the person or what they did and they will be able to connect it to him.

4 I consider an alternative reading of this scene in the next data analysis that involves the lost boys being doubles for the Surf Nazis, and that the attack on the vampires in the abandoned hotel is an attack on them.

5

DISCUSSION 1

The Oedipus complex in reputation, authority, and ambition

Although most people associate the Oedipus complex with the idea of "killing your father and fucking your mother," or with castration, this is not entirely accurate. The actual parents do not have to be involved, nor does sex, nor the threat of death or castration, nor does the third party have to be an actual person. We have seen that Sam's Oedipus complex involves his mother, Lucy, and a would-be suitor, Max, but that its structure came from the triangle of Michael, Star, and David, who do not have familial ties. My interest here is to turn to psychoanalytic theory to show how the Oedipus complex can be operationalized in several different ways in order to find the best way to understand the one that affects Sam in the latent plot.

The Oedipus complex, for Freud, is both a hypothesized childhood event, of which he conceives in both phylogenetic and ontogenetic terms, and a functional relation to authority and love figures in a person's life. I will return to the first conceptualization much later on, and begin with the latter. The Oedipus complex and its ties to love, as when a pattern of infidelity shows up in several, if not all, of someone's relationships (i.e. an "injured third party"), or when a woman has "daddy issues" and goes for emotionally distant men who are like her father, still show up in an occasional journal article to this day (Freud, 1910). However, it is more than just "family romances" that are hypothesized to be repetitions of relations to caregivers or siblings in childhood. Freud (1914b) writes:

> [W]e can now understand our relation to our schoolmasters. These men, not all of whom were in fact fathers themselves, became our substitute fathers. That was why, even though they were still quite young, they struck us as so mature and so unattainably adult. We transferred on to them the respect and expectations attaching to the omniscient father of our childhood, and we then began to treat them as we treated our fathers at home.

> We confronted them with the ambivalence that we had acquired in our own families and with its help we struggled with them as we had been in the habit of struggling with our fathers.
>
> *(p. 244)*

Our parents or caregivers provide us with not only models of love, but also of authority. Authority figures are seen as more perfect and in command of more experience, knowledge, and skill. Just as we encounter rules, threats of punishment, and expectations for performance in the home, we later find these in society as well, and we expand the circle of adults to whom we confer authority. Problems with authority within the home can also lead individuals to have problems with authority outside of the home (at various levels of society), but this ambivalence to a teacher, the police, a boss, etc., is not a given. I will return to this point of ambivalence vs. non-ambivalence again later, but for now I want to stress that Freud sees humans as eminently social animals.

In Freud's model of mind, he views humans as primarily related, and not as atomistic or primarily separated, rational agents. When Freud (1921) writes that only under "exceptional conditions" can psychology "disregard the relations of the individual to others," psychopathology like psychosis is what he has in mind (p. 69). The psychotic person can live in an eternal present in which they are catatonically alone, or they can be ambulatory and tell all those who will listen around them about the end of the world, the millions of dollars they used to have, or the help they need to locate their child (who has been deceased for years). This individual displays a regression from "the social drives," or ego and object drives, and either displays an apathy instead of a desire for connection with others, or demonstrates that there they make little to no differentiation between people (1911a, 1911b, 1914a, 1915a, 1917a, 1917c, 1920, 1930, 1933).[1] Compared to people who show very differentiated social drives and transferences, the self-absorbed ambulatory person with psychosis behaves as though his delusion is so important that all others need to hear about it. There are also examples of autistic children who never developed to more relatedness with others but instead remain completely dependent on their parents and find most of their interest in the inanimate environment or stereotyped gestures and movements.

The concept of the social drives is linked to psychic bisexuality and a horizontal axis in the economics of libido. Freud (1923a) perceives "two sets of emotional impulses . . . opposed to each other . . . impulses of an affectionate and submissive nature, but also hostile and defiant ones" (p. 85). Freud (1905, 1914a, 1924, 1930, 1933) aligns the female sex with passivity, submissiveness, and masochism in some places, and cautions against doing so in other places. In his late work, he laments that "we cannot but feel it as a serious impediment in psychoanalysis that it [bisexuality] has not yet found any link with the theory of the instincts" (Freud, 1930, p. 105 fn). However, in *The Economics of Libido* (2015) I argue that Freud does offer us a link in his remarks on the contrast between egoism and altruism in the motivations of people (Freud, 1913, 1917c, 1930). Very simply, there are active-egoistic people who are more power-based as evidenced in their competitiveness, desire to be admired, and ambition. In contrast, there are passive-altruistic people who are belonging-based and more cooperative, who desire to be in harmony with others, and who avoid conflict and are more engaged in empathy. There is evidence of active-egoistic and passive-altruistic drives in both primary masculinity and primary femininity and, because of psychic bisexuality, a biological male can express either active or passive feminine drives (and vice versa). Due to the complexity of this material, I will focus on the active-egoistic pole and the vertical axis of the superego to sketch an initial model of mind, and wait until the next book to develop the horizontal axis.

Freud gives us a type of drive psychology in which every social relation, as well as every narcissistic one, is related to a prototypical relation with a parent or sibling figure that forms an imago during psychosexual development. Although there are some cases in which the *personalized* beginnings of the drive and imago show up later in life (i.e. one's romantic partner has the same name as one's mother, similar eyes or appearance, or is close to her age), the *depersonalized* aspects are the most important (Freud, 1926a, p. 139; 1930, pp. 124–125; 1914a, p. 94). The latter aspect reflects how "a child has a different estimate of its parents at different periods of its life" and how these representations of parental power that are formed throughout psychosexual development correspond to different estimates of authority (Freud, 1933, p. 64). I will return to depersonalization shortly, but would like to continue to make a couple remarks about the "exceptional conditions" in which we are not driven to interact with other humans.

Drives are very fluid and can change their objects drastically. For example, one patient who had previously been driven to be a passive-altruistic "people-pleaser" or "helper" with others, felt taken for granted by people. She began removing herself from contact with others so that she did not have to face up to her inability to say no. However, I noticed that she was still able to satisfy this drive through her cats and plants. She would tell me stories about bringing a wilted plant back to health or making up stories about the cats in which they would be taught lessons of harmony and love, and I began to see that these stories ended that way in contrast to her past relations with men and friends, which did not have good endings. I have also worked with patients who play out dramas of authority and control with their pets, which are interesting idiosyncrasies when compared to their passive relations with people, as well as patients who have active relations with others, but who are very loving and nurturing with their pets. In contrast to the regression in psychosis, this type of example is closer to the concept of sublimation since these people still show functioning at higher levels of development.[2]

In a more classical example of sublimation, Freud (1917c) describes the process as the transferring of social drives through the introverted act of fantasying:

> [A]n artist is once more in rudiments an introvert, not far removed from neurosis. He is oppressed by excessively powerful instinctual needs. He desires to win honor, power, wealth, fame and the love of women; but he lacks the means for achieving these satisfactions. Consequently, like any other unsatisfied man, he turns away from reality and *transfers all his [ego] interest, and his [object] libido too, to the wishful constructions of his life of phantasy*, whence the path might lead to neurosis.
>
> *(p. 375, emphasis added)*

The social drives can be divided into ego (work and public life) and object (love and private life) manifestations. These in turn can be routed through earlier narcissistic or introverted drives like fantasying so that they are satisfied in stories, songs, or novels instead of real life. Far from an exhaustive cataloguing of drives, Freud isolates specific ones like "rescuing" and shows that they can they can involve a love object as well as have an ego drive manifestation and be enacted with "the emperor, a king, or some other great man" (Freud, 1910, pp. 172–173). In a more contemporary example, the latter can be seen in how some academics find a lesser known or neglected philosopher or thinker to champion as having not receiving his due, and want to "rescue him from obscurity." In the internal world of the artist's fantasying, the drive of rescuing becomes "withdrawn from the influence of other people" in the external world and expressed through characters in his story. However, we can recognize that an author's stories, or a daydreamer's fantasies, can still be cliché, highly derivative, and show the influence of others in another sense, so this division should not be taken as absolute.

To catalogue the drives is a task that remains close to both common language and what I have mentioned as the horizontal axis of psychic bisexuality. If we are to leave general concepts like ego interest and power for more specific drives, then they must reference the language of motivations that we ascribe to ourselves and others.[3] If we take the drive of rescuing above, it is clear that this is a specific act that could have several motivations. Someone could rescue another out of love—they would even endanger their own life in the rescue and preservation of the beloved. Someone could rescue others to be a hero, thus exhibiting a desire to be looked up to. Someone could also rescue another out of a sense of duty to a team member, out of guilt and knowing that they would want the same if the situation were reversed, and any other common language motivation that can be found. Both egoistic and altruistic motivations, and different ideals of conscience, can coexist, or be in confluence, in one individual. "The social instincts," Freud (1913) writes, "are themselves derived from a combination of egoistic and erotic [altruistic] components into wholes of a special kind" (p. 73). These "wholes" are the qualitative aspect of phenomenology and the increasing attunement to feeling and motivational states in others, and their ambivalences, is tied to the idea of becoming wise.

The ego and object drives that are expressed in the external world are routed through the different estimates of authority/power in the human environment or social body. Freud is explicit that in "the Oedipus complex . . . [the parents'] personal significance for the superego recedes into the background" and "the imagos they leave behind . . . link [to] the influences of teachers and authorities" (Freud, 1924, pp. 167–168; 1919a, p. 190). The imago forms the superego, and the motivational ties to the perfection of authority are expressed in its ego-ideal aspect through a "double kind of tie . . . putting the object in the place of the ego ideal" (Freud, 1921, p. 130). "There is no doubt," Freud (1933) writes, "that this ego ideal is the precipitate of the old picture of the parents, the expression of admiration for the perfection which the child then attributed to them" (p. 65). Chasseguet-Smirgel (1976a, p. 282; 1976b, pp. 354, 358) conceptualizes this depersonalized aspect of the Oedipus complex as establishing the *difference between the generations*. So conceived, the difference between the generations can be recognized in any culture in which there are elders or leaders with more Prestige and neophytes who are held in lower esteem. On one hand, the esteem seems rational because the elders will have more experience and therefore skills or knowledge that the neophytes will want to learn. On the other hand, there is a tension between this formulation since Prestige is sometimes due to belonging to a higher class, caste, or "noble" family that has nothing to do with their skills or knowledge. A person can triangulate with both types, and will often transfer superiority in abilities or knowledge to those who occupy structural positions of power through their name or class.

The conceptualization of the different levels of authority has hitherto been something that has not been done well, or coherently, in psychoanalysis. In "Group Psychology and Analysis of the Ego" (1921), Freud writes of different ego ideals that we put on authority figures and love objects, but not in any formalized way. For example, the ego ideal that is put upon a hypnotist and results in him or her being able to plant thoughts into one's mind is a very primitive and powerful form of power (ibid., p. 125). Freud then compares the power of the hypnotist to the *mana* or power that primitive chiefs or kings had and thus an ego ideal that gives a transference to an authority who appears as semi-divine or magical is evidenced (ibid.). This felt power or perfection of the king, in turn, would differ from the ego ideal that one might put on a general or captain in the army and Freud discusses how leadership is necessary for soldiers to overcome their conscience or inhibitions of killing in war. This example opens up a whole other dimension of the superego in relation to group psychology and conscience that I will explore in the next chapter, but for the moment I want to stay with the thread of different levels of perfection/authority and the trait of ambition.

These different levels of the ego ideal are conscious, although sometimes preconscious, motivations that a person can avow. A patient can tell her therapist, for example, that she is enraged by her boyfriend watching pornography, and that she wants to be the only woman he desires, or that she knows that she is pretty, but that she feels like she should be as beautiful as models in magazines. Outside the clinic, popular culture often provides an athlete who is shameless enough to announce to the world that he is the greatest that there has ever been. An actor might quote the box office of their movies as evidence of why he should be regarded as first in his field despite his lack of an Oscar. Additionally, such ideals are sometimes expressed indirectly too by people without success. For example, a person may criticize every new book that comes out as if he had written a library full of them and thus had the authority to critique harshly. In such instances of grandiosity or arrogance, the psychodynamic formulation of the person having assumed the place of the parental imago or having become his ego ideal (as opposed to trying to live up to it) is an important operation.[4]

Wanting to be admired for one's skills or knowledge and to have a good reputation in the community is the phallic-oedipal form of the ego ideal. In contemporary cultures this can include wanting to be admired for one's computer skills, for example, but in a primitive political economy having skills for hunting, for example, might be the input for how a person might compete with others for reputation. The trait of ambition references going beyond one's community and registering in higher social hierarchies in which one seeks to be "the best."

However, ambition can still deepen past this point of wanting to be the best. The ambitious person may want to attain a level of being a name that is immortalized in history or to be "the best there ever was." Such an individual may feel tensions of inferiority, or self-criticism of the ego for not being an "immortal" writer like Shakespeare or Goethe, regardless of how much public success has already been garnered.

Freud (1914a) observes that just because someone has an ambitious ego ideal, this does not mean that he or she will have the power to sublimate and achieve the desired Prestige or authority. He writes:

> It is precisely in neurotics that we find the highest differences of potential between the development of their ego ideal and the amount of sublimation of their primitive libidinal instincts . . . the formation of an ideal heightens the demands of the ego and is the most powerful factor favouring repression. *(p. 95)*

Freud's point here is that more ambitious people will encounter frustration from bosses, teachers, those who are wealthier, those who have inherited influence or power, etc., and are more open to ego injuries from these parental-substitutes. Unless such a person has had the discipline to able to become very skilled in their field, has a good memory and is able to synthesize knowledge in another field, and all the other traits required to do important work, then he or she may encounter enough frustration to end up repressing this part of their personality or forming a neurotic symptom.[5] The likelihood of these outcomes is straightforward once one considers what someone who is competitive and driven to seek admiration or recognition for having superior knowledge, for example, will face.[6] The person goes from competing in primary school, middle school, and then getting a high school diploma, to a BA, to an MA, to a PhD. Prestige further defines ambition, thus even after the PhD, the ambitious person seeks additional Prestige through her publications and whether they secure a job at an ivy league school. However, even if one gets a good professorship and publishes, she may not be a luminary in the field. One can also be regarded as a luminary in the field, but still not be remembered or read much in a few generations. Becoming an immortal name, who will always be taught in the history of a discipline, or a world-historical individual, is still another level of attainment. If one can fathom the pressure on individuals with deep ambition, then both the anger and rage that will emerge in their frustration with the parental-substitutes or gatekeepers to these different levels, and its repression (in those of them who are not sociopaths) will make sense.

Outside of academia we are all familiar with personal or cultural examples of those who "become neurotic because [they] wanted to be something better than what, with [their] origin, [they] are capable of being" (Freud, 1908, p. 182). There is the talented athlete who got an injury and did not make it to "the big league" and became an alcoholic, the musician with ambition who did not make it, cannot reconcile himself to a normal job, and still "acts like a kid," or the local beauty who moved to a larger city to become famous and ends up moving back and becomes a shut-in. These clichés illustrate that the Oedipus complex is about being driven to find social satisfactions (of which admiration for skill, beauty, or knowledge is one example). It is also the idea that the ego injuries that people receive in social embarrassments or disappointments in love with parental-substitutes, will relate to repression and be the cause of psychopathology. While these kinds of narratives are well known, finer details are important in this formulation, and I will expand on them below.

I

I would like to quickly turn to the popular understanding of the superego, particularly for any readers who are scratching their head about the interpretation of the superego given so far. If one looks at almost any general textbook on psychology that includes a section on Freud, it will say that the superego will be characterized as that which deals with guilt and replaces the Oedipus complex, which emerges in the phallic stage of psychosexual development. I have shared some quotations that deal with the ego-ideal aspect of the superego, often neglected in the popular understanding, and now I will show how this version ignores two key aspects of Freud's work in the area of conscience.

The first is that the guilt conscience is actually formed in the phase after the Oedipus complex and is not universal. In the "New Introductory Lectures," Freud (1933) writes, "God has done an uneven and careless piece of work, for a large majority of men have brought along with them only a modest amount of [conscience], or scarcely enough to be worth mentioning" (p. 61). He identifies the post-oedipal phase of the full guilt conscience with interactions with siblings in what he calls *the father complex* (Freud, 1923b, p. 37). Moreover, he explicitly links the Oedipus complex to what he calls *social anxiety* in differentiation from the father complex (Freud, 1926a, p. 139). Regarding the latter, he writes:

> [I]n many adults . . . the place of the father or the two parents is taken by the larger human community . . . such people habitually allow themselves to do any bad thing which promises them enjoyment, so long as they are sure that the authority will not know anything about it or cannot blame them for it; they are afraid only of being found out.
>
> *(Freud, 1930, pp. 124–125)*

Social anxiety stands in stark contrast to the subsequent guilt conscience, in which the individual may judge himself as bad for what he intends to do, or feels like he must come clean about his misdeeds in order to be OK with himself (Freud, 1930, p. 131). As Freud points out, social anxiety can be tied to an individual's bad conscience that amounts to remorse after the deed, but this does not necessarily translate into internal pressure to tell someone how you wronged them (ibid.).[7] Guilt is about a sense of equality with others, which generates fairness and *social feeling*; social anxiety concerns one's reputation as a good person in the community or public (Freud, 1921, p. 121; 1923b, p. 37). Historically, there is a game of honor that comprises the ethical life in a given political economy. Within it, definitions of what a good person is required to do, or is prohibited from doing, are given. A person may play it without having her own scruples and therefore have no problem doing what is prohibited when she thinks the public, or important people in her life, will not find out.[8] Thus, the bridge between the superego as shame conscience and as the ego ideal's "demand for ever greater perfection" is in the importance of reputation. One can be shamed by others looking down on one for doing something regarded as ethically bad, but also be shamed about being viewed as weak, pathetic, or "sucking" at something in one's work life or hobbies. The bridge of reputation in these two areas also makes sense of the use of "good" in both ethical and work spheres. One can be "good" in the sense of being good at one's profession, studies, or job, for example, and also be good in an ethical sense of following rules, being respectful, and fair. Like ambition, there are qualitatively different levels of transgression in ethical life that we can see in common language expressions like someone violating something sacred and being evil or monstrous, to something illegal or "criminal" like stealing, to something more mundane like a faux pas. I will take this up in the next chapter when I talk about group psychology, but for the moment I want to stay with the internal aspects of the self-criticism of the superego.

The superego mediates transference to external objects, but the imago that comprises the superego also has other qualities that may be associated with it. In its external aspect, I have sketched the sense of different levels in society, and how common language expresses the magnitude of the different levels. The very general term "inferiority" can reference feeling "less than" or incompetent, but also grow in magnitude to feeling like a "bum," "a nobody," "a total loser" or a "complete nothing" as some patients have put it. However, along with these different levels there are compulsive symptoms ("dictatorial thou shalts") such as compulsive scheduling, compulsive working, and other expressions of the imagos' perfection (Freud, 1923b, pp. 54–55).

In such symptoms, the ego function or type of cognition associated with the psychosexual stage of development of a particular imago, comes into prominence. Although there is anxiety related to not completing the compulsive symptom, self-criticism and judgment also occur when something is not as clean as it should be, or when things are not going according to schedule.

I would like to begin to complicate this sketch a little more by returning to the idea of ambivalence and non-ambivalence with authority figures. We all can note many possible relationships with teachers or bosses. Some students in grad school, for example, are defiant and insinuate that their professors do not understand the work under discussion (and usually are much more defamatory at the bar after class). Other students idealize their professors and need to speak with them after class and have some kind of personal relationship with them in which they feel their approval—some of whom wish to continue their advisor's work and add to his or her legacy. As with our parents, our own names may become attached to our advisor's name and appear on papers with theirs. They may give us a pedigree in academia, and we may be caught up with their reputation or image, and they may be caught up in ours.

This relation of having one's name caught up with one's family of origin, or with a pedigree in one's work life, is the best way to conceptualize the (phallic) Oedipus complex. In my work with addicts, there are many who began using as teenagers and one can often quickly obtain from them when they stopped caring about their grades in school and about wanting to make their parents proud. From another angle, this can be ascertained negatively from when they no longer cared about embarrassing their parents, became indifferent to their teachers' opinions about them, and became part of the "wrong crowd," "the rejects," or risked criminal charges for selling drugs. At this point, such patients show that they regressed from caring about what will give them a bad reputation and will often talk about seeking acceptance by hanging out with the other "bad kids" or joining gangs, for example. On their own, and without reconstruction, some of them can quite specifically bring up events with their actual parents that made them "not care anymore," while others recount severe bullying, or some other blow to their ego.

To return to the example of grad students, what is important is that we can acknowledge that not everyone is defiant, submissive, ingratiating, etc., with their professor or advisor. Some people can take authority into their ego ideal in a way that is non-ambivalent, in which there is *Eros* or fusion with the parental imagoes. They are given respect, even if one can see some shortcomings, and one tries to learn what one can from them. Some will defuse from the imago or have a relation of *Phobos*, in which there is a distance from the parental imago and relations with parental-substitutes show signs of ambivalence. Acknowledging this difference, I began considering the "complex" of the Oedipal situation as that which refers to whatever causes defusion or the Phobos relation with the imago (Pederson, 2015). In contrast, I use the term castration complex to refer to the many different repetitions with authority figures, lovers, and friends in which the ambivalence produces anxiety situations. I will have some clinical examples of some ambivalent relations a little later on.

As mentioned in the first data analysis, the Oedipus complex also compromises that the child recognizes that the mother wants love in an adult relationship and could not be satisfied by a relationship with a child (Chasseguet-Smirgel 1976a, p. 282). There is a parallel between the child recognizing someone with superior skill or knowledge in the paternal imago and the difference between the generations with the mother belonging with the father. There is a caveat I will make to this a little later on, but what is important for the moment is that Freud (1921) also uses the ego ideal to denote the idealization of the love object in the sphere of the object drives (p. 113). At the phallic Oedipus complex, Freud holds that the active boy is capable of full anaclitic love, which is characterized as "affectionate," although at earlier stages there can still be infatuation/idealization with the sexual object (Freud, 1921, p. 111; 1923b, p. 32).

The centrality of the phallic castration complex is that it represents the pinnacle of striving for happiness in work life, love life, and synthesis in friendship. There is a parallelism between the ego drive and the object drive. Just as an active-egoist may be possessive of his "girl," or jealous of the attractive partners of peers, he can also be possessive regarding his reputation as competent or being among the intelligent or skilled at work and be "jealous" of another's promotion. Besides being passed over for a raise, Freud (1911b) alerts us to how "mishap[s] in social relations with other men" in general can cause embarrassment, shame, or mortifications that will dam up or intensify the libido (p. 62). This social anxiety, along with the anxiety of having one's moral reputation ruined in the community, is often connected to one's reputation as a man or woman. In running different therapy groups, I have heard one male member admonish another for not "handling things like a man" or being a "little bitch." This is the much better known "difference between the sexes" of the Oedipus complex. It recognizes the input of gender in relation to being shamed socially. It is also seen as a node for pathology in different intrapsychic operations that allow a man who has been hurt in love, for example, to become a misogynist and defensively represent women as bad, weak, or troublesome.

The last important input, one that we actually see in the myth of Oedipus, is the relation to oneself in promise-making. Shame can also be something one feels in relation to oneself (i.e. "I am ashamed of myself") and breaking a promise (i.e. "a man's word is his bond") is a good example of the cause of such shame.[9] I have also worked with many men who have had to "forgive themselves" for losing their wealth, family, for not realizing their ambitions, or for some of the lies that they told. In the myth, Oedipus has *hubris* for making his promise to find whoever is responsible for the plague in Thebes. The moral seems to be that one should not make grand promises, lest one be unable to fulfill them and lose face in front of others or lose self-respect (i.e. be ashamed of oneself). Promises can be taken as a self-prohibition included in the conscience aspect of the superego, but as mentioned above, promise-making is different than forming the full guilt conscience of the father complex, and feeling oneself to be equal to others.

I would like to give a clinical example of this relation to oneself:

> Client has associations that lead us to his feelings of shame. I ask him to sit with the feeling and then tell me other times in the past he remembers feeling like this. Client tells me that he remembers the first time in jail, when he relapsed for a second time with a girlfriend he had promised he'd be better to, and even all the way back to a run in with a police officer when he was a pre-teen. Client tells me that he feels it in his shoulders and chest and expresses it as the feeling that he'll be "thrown away."
>
> We go to his first DUI, before he had any serious time in jail. Client begins to feel the shame expand to his face and it combines with a feeling of "helplessness." He stays with it as I do more BLS and anger soon begins to come in quite strongly. I ask him who he feels it towards and he and says "myself." I tell him that he needs to discharge it and that he should picture his younger self in jail and tell this self how he's screwing up his life and to verbalize the anger as much as he can. I add that if words aren't enough and if he feels that his body wants to physically express itself, that he should go further. I begin BLS and after a few minutes he signals me to stop. He tells me that he yelled at himself and ended up punching and then putting himself in "a choke hold" until this self had told him that he would listen. However, client doesn't feel like all the somatic tension is gone (although he reports that it has been reduced a good amount). I know there is a second part to this and I point out that he's the one who has made those future decisions to relapse and squander his youth and not this younger self. I ask him if he can flip this script and if he can ask this self for forgiveness for what he's done? He looks at me intently, and nods his head, yes. I begin BLS and he again goes for several minutes before signaling me.
>
> Spontaneously he begins to tell me that he apologized for not listening to others who told him the right things to do, for doing what he wanted to do, and thinking that he knew everything. Client says that he apologized for putting his younger self through all he had put him through and that afterwards this self "looked understanding." He adds that he "thanked him for sticking it out and not giving up completely," and that he owned up to being "hardheaded and stubborn." Lastly, client adds that he eventually learned right and wrong. I ask him to focus on the look of understanding that this self had, and to see if his body has any reaction to it, as he pictures it. I begin BLS and after a few moments he nods to signal a change going on and I continue for a few moments until he signals that it's done. He says that his younger self "looked more comfortable in his cell" and he expresses that his shoulder and chest tension have released and he feels very relaxed. I ask him to float back to another time he felt like this and he tells me that it was on a golf course with his father. He adds that it's a cloudy day and that he has always loved cloudy days. He says he feels extremely comfortable and like he has no responsibility, like a kid.

In this example, my patient's anger became focused on himself and not a parental-substitute. He was unhappy with where he ended up in life and after discharging his anger, an apology to himself was needed to process the relation to his self imago. Thus, whether it is a triangular relation to failing oneself in regards to success, love, or friendship, breaking a promise, or an ethical transgression, the anxiety and/or shame is a pivot point for defensive operations.

I would like to give another example in which such a defensive operation is in place, but this time the focus will be more about the relation to the imago as that which imbues one with both maturational (i.e. difference between the generations) and masculine qualities (i.e. difference between the sexes):

> Client begins the session by telling me that we need to talk about his stepfather. He initially paints a picture of how things were good between them and that there were "family trips," they would go to the shooting range together, there were family BBQs at the park, and how he'd come to client's baseball games. He mentions "projects" and how his stepfather taught client to build a dog house, and other things, and I get a sense for the fullness he had in his life. But when his stepfather and mother divorced when client was age 16, he tells me that his stepfather "changed, he became a complete asshole." I ask client for the lead up to the divorce and he tells me that his stepfather got into an accident at his job, wasn't able to work, and fell into depression. He tells me that his mother stood by his stepfather for as long as she could, but as his stepfather isolated himself further and got "meaner," she eventually left him. Client tells me that he was allowed to pick who he'd live with and he chose his stepfather because he "wasn't going to leave him alone." Client tells me that he started working to help support him and dropped out of high school. Client tells me how his stepfather got a bit better and returned to work himself, but that he would "fly off the handle" and "say fucked up things to [him]." Client gives me a few instances, which culminated in a time when his stepfather told him that he was "not [his] son." I can tell that client gives this a lot of gravity and I see how important it was that his brother stood up for him and said that if client wasn't his son, that he wasn't his father's son either. Client admits that it "hurt [his] feelings" and "there's a part of [him] that's never lived it down." Client also registers some surprise at the feelings and shares how he thought that he had "moved past it."
>
> Client goes on to talk about their other fights, and I get the sense that he wants me to understand more, so I don't get him to stop at this ego injury. He comes back to it on his own a few times, and expresses that his stepfather was "the person he least expected to say messed up stuff to [him]." He lets me know that after it happened, that he had thought to himself "do what you're going to do and I'll do me." Client reports he went to live on his own, but that he moved back in with his stepfather several times. He tells me that he was using a lot of drugs at this time and strangely the narrative begins to change from his stepfather "the asshole" to the stepfather who tried

to "get [him] to snap out of [his] addiction." Client talks about the "advice and warnings" his stepfather would give him and how client "didn't listen to him." I confront client with these two representations of his stepfather, since the new one is so different than the previous one. However, he acknowledges them both and does not seem troubled by them.

I ask client to focus on his "asshole" stepfather and the stepfather who tried to help him but didn't know how to reach him. I ask him to see which one he has a bigger reaction to and begin BLS. Client reports that it is the latter and reports that he feels it very strongly in his chest. I ask client to see what his body wants to do and resume BLS. He reports that it gets a bit tighter in his chest but then it stops. I ask him to project it out. He tells me that he sees a rope "pulled tight." I ask him what kind of rope he pictured and he says a "towing rope." I ask him for the first association to a towing rope and brings up a time his car "took a shit on him" and his stepfather showed up to tow him. He tells me that it's a good memory. I ask him to see if he can introject the rope into his chest. He tells me that he can and gestures that it fits in vertically during BLS. Client reports afterwards that he feels like he's "calmed down" some, but otherwise he doesn't have a reaction to the rope in his body or mind. I return him to the representation of his stepfather trying to help him and he now gets in touch with sadness, and I see tears in his eyes. I remind him that he's a man now but that if this 16-year-old self needs to come in to him and let out what he held in at the time, that client needs to have compassion for him. Client's sadness doesn't deepen, instead he begins to tell me about when he learned that his stepfather wasn't his real father as a boy and how client got "a chip on his shoulder." He says that he both wanted to "be left alone" and "get attention." He says that he "pushed [his family] away" but would also be "snotty, selfish," and "used [his] hurt as an excuse to act out." He tells me that sometimes only his brother could talk him down.

After detailing how his parents would "finally get tired of [his] shit" and let him get away with things, he returns to the age of 16. Instead of choosing to live with his father, so that he wasn't alone, Client now tells me that he "knew [he]'d get out of going to school" and that "[he]'d have to work" if he went with his stepfather. Client expresses that he went with his stepfather because he had still been "childish," but that he "finally started to mature" and his stepfather had tried "to show [him] how to be responsible." I ask client what happened, and what stopped him from listening to his stepfather's lessons. Client tells me that he "couldn't measure up to [his stepfather]" and "didn't want to fail trying." He tells me that he's had a "fear of failure" since he was age 12. He tells me that this is when his mother first caught him getting high. He told me that his stepfather "smacked [his] ass" but client "laughed it off"; he submitted to the punishments but would never show that they hurt him. He tells me that he just "learned to be more sneaky" and that if he was "a complete asshole . . . they would leave [him] alone . . . so they didn't have to deal with [him] or hear [him]." Client goes on to explain how he "wanted to fit in and hang out with the older crowd" when he was 12. Being an insider with the cool crowd was important to him and school didn't feel important, so when client chose to move in with his stepfather at 16, he wanted to be grown up and older but soon learned it was "not fun." Client tells me about the fights he and his stepfather got in at this time and how his stepfather would tell client how the world is and how one day client "will have his own family, work every day, and know what it's about." Client looks at me and says, "Fuck, dad was right."

Client tells me about how he got laid off from his job at that time and that they never hired him back when they took back some of his coworkers. Client admits that he was "an asshole" at work, just like he was with his family. He tells me that this is when he decided to "make fast money" and sold meth. He details how he made his fast money, used too much of the meth himself, and how he was back and forth with moving out and returning to his stepfather. Client reports his stepfather still tried to "help [him] see" and "learn to be a man," but also saw that client had to want to change himself and told client that he had "to pull [him]self up." This culminated with client joining a gang in his mid twenties. He's able to express to me how they became his "new family" and client "fully backed away from [his] stepfather." Client explains that things were "superficial" when they would talk after this point. Client tells me that one time a friend of his stepfather's told him that client "wasn't doing right" and was going to get into "serious trouble." This led to client's stepfather pressing the issue and they got into a fistfight. Client reports that they didn't talk for months afterwards and that when they finally did, his stepfather expressed that he felt like he "failed [him] as a father." His stepfather went on to say that he "didn't want to outlive his child." Client looks at me very intently at this point and says that his stepfather "was insinuating that he was failing [him] . . . but all this happened because [*he*] was afraid of failure."

This strikes me as another important moment with client. I ask him to take what he's told me about his fear of failure and not being able to measure up to his stepfather, being an asshole and pushing others away, and everything else, and to picture his stepfather at age 16 and to tell him everything he couldn't say back then in his mind's eye. After BLS, I ask client how his stepfather took it and client says that he said "it's normal to be scared son, it's healthy . . . it'll all come in time." Client then reports that the representation told him that he had tried to make client "strong for the world." Client is saying this in a new tone of voice and I can tell something is changing. I ask him to continue picturing his stepfather speaking to him like this and resume BLS. I find myself telling client during this that "he already has everything it takes to be man." After, client tells me that he feels "relaxed" and feels "comfort" in his chest. I ask him to focus on the well-being and to tell me when he remembers feeling like this in the past, and he tells me at his grandma's house as a kid. He details what it was like to have a "sleepover" there, and I instill the memory of when he "was little."

In this example, we see that my patient initially defended against his failure of maturation by projecting his "asshole" attitude onto his stepfather. This is not to say that his stepfather had not been out of line with some of the things he had told his son, but only that my patient had changed the narrative and described himself with the same word. As many other patients do, he represented this lack of maturation as him being a "kid" and as a lack of manliness/masculinity.

The fact that he had brought this material into the session himself and had hinted about his "fear of failure" in earlier sessions, points to how we might regard the figure of Tiresias in the Oedipus myth as a double of Oedipus. Just as Tiresias knows the truth about the cause of the plague, my patient had known about how he had failed his stepfather, had been the cause of their "superficial" relationship, and turned to "fast money" and power out of fear and inferiority feelings.

This clinical example, which showcases my patient's regression from his caring about reputation and family, to criminality, a new crime family, and addiction, brings up one more important distinction concerning the phallic Oedipus complex. While every normal child (ex. excluding children in developmental arrest) has reached the phallic Oedipus complex, there is an important difference between the narcissistic individual who has not gone on to further development of the superego in latency and the neurotic who has reached latency.[10] The narcissistic individual may regress to where he can no longer work or love, while the neurotic individual has a post-ambivalent tie to society. In Freud's account, there is a further development of the superego in latency (Freud, 1926a, p. 142). The child goes on to form an *identity-ego* in which the post ambivalent tie to culture is mediated by group minds: "those of his race, of his class, of his creed, of his nationality, etc." (Freud, 1921, p. 129). These group minds are also objects for the narcissists who have not formed the latency superego, but they are always ambivalent and tied to parental imagos in such cases. Psychoanalysts like Vamik Volkan (1997) study the interaction of group minds and self-esteem under the heading of "large group narcissism," but these ideas will not be part of my analysis since the films are focused on individual narcissism. I have included them to help my reader get more context for the Freudian model of the personality.

Before I offer further refinements to the model of mind that I have sketched, I would like to give a summary and more exposition to the role of the imago in its object drive expression. So far, we have seen that there is the *depersonalized* aspect of the parental imagos that allow for parental-substitutes to be put in the ego ideal for both ego and object drives, and that registers their authority/power/idealization at levels of deepening and greater magnitude. In the object drives, or the energy that pushes toward a romantic relationship, these levels can be shown when patients report that they feel their partner is "out of their league," and they wonder why he or she is interested in him. It can also be seen in "class climbing" through romantic relationships or marriage in which attraction follows partners of more Prestige, wealth, or perceived quality.

The depersonalized imago is also connected to the difference between the sexes and how object-choice (both sexual and love feelings) becomes heterosexual.

Classically, Freud and others have strangely speculated that the boy gets to keep the mother as object, while the girl has to change. I see no evidence for this, and instead have proposed that in the difference between the generations both boy and girl recognize the father possessing the mother as a template of complementarity that both girl and boy must follow.[11] The mother, or primary parent, is the first object for both boy and girl (Freud, 1938a, p. 155). Even if the primary parent is a man with a bottle there is an instinct that a child is born with for the breast/nipple that associates the primary parent with the breast. As I will return to later, the father is not naturally superior, but receives his symbolic position as the *not-mother*, which means that the breast will be replaced by the phallus and that there is an underlying "equation" of the two (Klein, 1932, pp. 213–214). This structural, maternal, and paternal relation of the imago continues even if one's father stays at home and mother works, or one has two mothers, for example. This is not to say that non-traditional families will have no influence on one's character, because analysts like Stoller (1976) have shown this in some cases. Rather, the point is that power differences between the parents, whether gay or straight, will register in the maternal and paternal structure, on one hand. On the other, studies show that having same-sex parents does not produce gay or lesbian children at the same frequency that opposite-sex parents produce straight children. This indicates that the actual sex of the parents is not as important as the structural relation of the maternal and paternal imagos and the nature and nurture influences in early psychosexual stages.

This form of the imago can be contrasted to the *transpersonalized* internal object or phantasy version of the imago. The term internal object was used by Klein (1932, 1935, 1940, 1975) and concerns how a phantasy representation of an imago can show up in play, stories, or cultural representations, as well as dreams, fantasies, or associations in the clinic. A witch, for example, can be a representation of a bad imago (i.e. bad internal object), that relates to a primitive level of development in which the parents are believed to have magical or very great powers. The witch may want to "gobble up children," and this shows the tie to a specific id form of aggression.[12] Id impulse, bodily zone, and associated products (ex. the voice, feces, urine) influence the phantastic form, but also remain something separate or separable from it. Beyond mere representation of the internal maternal and paternal structure of the imagos, their phantastic aspect would correspond to Jungian archetypes and enduring representations of mother earth and father sky, for example.

I have also mentioned the *personalized* aspect of the imago and would also like to talk about the possible *repersonalized* dimension of the imago. In the personalized aspect, a man's choice of woman might resemble his mother, his father, a sibling, etc., in some features of her appearance, her gait, her interests, in some parts of her identity, or her style. In Chapter 2 we saw how narcissistic object-choice can register such dimensions concerning oneself, and the same can apply to a parent in anaclitic object-choice. I have had several borderline patients who have referenced the similarity in appearance, name, or age between their partners and parents on their own, without any prompting from me. In contrast, it is also clear that many patients stay close to their actual parents to help regulate their self-esteem and mental illness.

The parents repeat the roles they took in the patient's childhood and become a powerful authority figure who must be obeyed or controlled, or completely responsible for one, or requiring one's help. This is what I term a repersonalized imago. If the individual is not too self-absorbed and still has social ties or object constancy in work, love, and friendships, then this often appears as the child becoming an adult who has become the friend of one of, or both parents. If the person is low-functioning, then this can appear as "the 40-year-old virgin" who lives at home with his mother. In the latter case, there is an unconscious repersonalized imago relationship with his mother with the sexual feelings being unconscious (except in extreme cases). In contrast, in the depersonalized form, a man might be on his third or fourth marriage with a parental-substitute for whom he has conscious sexual feelings.

II

At this point I would like to introduce further refinements to Freud's model of mind, which I did not offer in *The Economics of Libido* (2015). So far, I have introduced the ego ideal under the auspices of an active-egoistic motivational structure that relates to competition, ambition, and power. The ego ideal determines the level of a person's ambition and "demands perfection," or that one live up to this level, or face inferiority tensions and jealousy/envy regarding others. However, Freud (1914a) also introduces the ego ideal as having an aspect relating to "self-regard" (pp. 98–100), which he later clarifies in *Group Psychology and Analysis of the Ego* (1921), by noting that

> the individual gives up his ego ideal and substitutes for it the group ideal as embodied in the leader . . . [but in] many individuals the separation between the ego and the ego ideal is not very far advanced; the two still coincide readily; *the ego has often preserved its earlier narcissistic self-complacency*. The selection of the leader is very much facilitated by this circumstance. He need often only possess the typical qualities of the individuals concerned in a particularly clearly marked and pure form, and need only *give an impression of greater force and of more freedom of libido*; and in that case the need for a strong chief will often meet him half-way and invest him with a predominance to which he would otherwise perhaps have had no claim. The other members of the group, whose ego ideal would not, apart from this, have become embodied in his person without some correction, are then carried away with the rest by "suggestion," that is to say, by means of identification.
>
> *(pp. 129–130, emphasis added)*

Freud's point here is best spelled out by saying that some people "naturally" inspire others as leaders because they have taken back some of the idealization of the parental imago. Those with less of an ego ideal, have both an increased self-regard and a decreased imperative to measure themselves by comparing their competency or experience to that of others.

In common language, this is simply a comment on confidence being attractive in those who have it. Confidence is different than vanity, arrogance, or cockiness and can be distinguished from the self-esteem of average people who don't have it. "A man who has been the indisputable favorite of his mother," Freud famously writes, "keeps for life the feeling of a conqueror, that confidence of success that often induces real success" (Jones, 1953, p. 5). In some ways, this also follows the popular cynicism that the people who often get into positions of power are seldom those who are the most hardworking, the most intelligent, or skilled. Rather, they usually feel entitled to be in those positions and can inspire others to have a similar confidence in them. The person with a full or high ego ideal has to earn self-esteem through performance and conscientiousness. He or she worries about being judged as incompetent and wants to make a good impression on the boss. However, I do not want to merely define this as deficiency since it can make a virtue of risk-taking and not following the traditional route in a way that is sometimes valuable. In parallel, this issue of confidence is readily apparent when it comes to the opposite sex. For example, confidence can be seen in how some men can approach women they do not know, while others fear rejection or compensate by boasting or name-dropping. All the vicissitudes of self-esteem are readily observable in both work and love life.

In Wilhelm Reich's work this dual notion of a high ego ideal and low ego ideal is noted. In regards to the former, Reich (1990) writes:

> Since a more or less conscious feeling of impotence is always present, many social accomplishments are primarily compensatory proofs of potency. These accomplishments, however, do not diminish the feelings of inferiority. On the contrary . . . the neurotic character never rids himself of the feeling of inner emptiness and incapacity, no matter how arduously he tries to compensate for it. Thus, the positive demands of the ego-ideal are raised higher and higher, while the ego, powerless and doubly paralyzed by feelings of inferiority (impotency and high ego-ideal), becomes less efficient.
>
> *(p. 180)*

This high ego ideal and the demand for "high and higher" achievements is contrasted to the "cocky" and "self-assured" phallic-narcissistic type who feels like he should be in a leading role or that he does not have to prove himself as much (ibid., pp. 123, 217–218). Reich also talks about the "impressive bearing" of phallic-narcissistic character (ibid., p. 217). Like Freud, he sees that those with a low ego ideal can inspire the transference to a parental-substitute without necessarily having the Prestige from accreditation (i.e. a degree) or money, nor from having demonstrated superior skill or knowledge in a contest. Interestingly, those who carried on Reich's characterology replaced the phallic-narcissistic character with the rigid or industrious/over-focused character that exemplifies the high ego ideal (Lowen, 1994; Kurtz, 2007). Lowen (1994) also introduces what he calls a "psychopathic" character that may have been meant to replace the phallic-narcissistic in some ways, but he does not identify it with the phallic stage, but an earlier one. I will return to this when I later differentiate the phallic from the anal and earlier forms of the superego in the next chapter. Lastly, Reich (1990) links phallic-narcissistic character to the symbol of the phallic mother, which is an important bridge for other accounts (p. 222).[13]

Ernest Jones' (1933) makes an important differentiation between the proto and deutero phallic phases that also seems to capture this distinction. However, as with much classical psychoanalysis, it focuses exclusively on the sexual, without reference to the ego drives. His observation is that this phase "is more self-centered, the chief allo-erotic attribute still remaining being its exhibitionistic aspect. It is thus less aggressive and less related to other people" (ibid., p. 4). Jones also sees that there is a higher proclivity to perversion, more interest in the penis, less connection to women, and more overt fantasies of success or power. Although Jones' focus is more on pathology, I find it important for two reasons. First, he links the deutero phase to Klein's concept of a combined parental imago, one example of which is the phallic mother that Reich observed (Klein, 1975). Second, his terms allow us to get away from the overly burdened term of narcissism, avoiding the confusion this term brings. Third, his usage allows me to coin the term trito to reference the post-oedipal father complex at other stages (i.e. phallic trito, anal trito, etc.).

McDougall (1972) sees what is effectively a deutero phase arising by the mother splitting the paternal imago that will become the oedipal father and creating a rival phallic image. "[S]he denigrates the father's phallic function . . . [and] gives the child in addition the feeling that he or she is a phallic substitute," McDougall (1972) writes, "another model of virility [which] was held up to the child, sometimes the mother's own father, or brother, sometimes a religious figure, or God is the one phallic object of value" (p. 381). McDougall is not the only analyst who has noted the phallic mother producing a different type of ego ideal. For example, Lampl-De Groot (1952) has also found this connection. "[T]he boy's ego-ideal," she writes, "had been selected originally in accordance with the example of the mother (although it was the phallic mother)" (p. 341). However, McDougall's phenomenology of this has been the most helpful to me. In her case study in "The Anonymous Spectator" (1974), she captures very strongly how the phallic image influenced her patient's perverse sexual relationship through the image of his grandfather chasing his mother with a whip in hand. She also details his ego drives and castration anxiety:

> "[T]o be like the others" still signified castration, "to be accepted by the others" was equivalent to losing his identity. He would then be forced to go over to the other side, the side of the brothers—and the fathers. To make such a move would mean the risk of losing all hope of possessing the mother's phallic secret and thus one day possessing the means of totally satisfying her . . . The Oedipal situation with its accompanying anxieties had never been faced, simply circumvented. This was achieved largely through two major defenses—disavowal and the disguise of "play." These served to deny

> the primal scene through inventing a counterfeit couple and also to convert castration anxiety into its opposite by treating it as a game . . . Deprived of the solution which allows identification with the father, he sees himself as the object of his mother's desire and her true complement. He comes to believe he can avoid the human sexual dilemma. He gets the diploma without passing the examination. But this is his bitter reward—he keeps it on condition that he never uses it. Nevertheless the fraudulent diploma, stolen from a repudiated father . . . [makes him a] paper king with an imitation scepter, [and] he must thereafter protect this identity and convince the others that his illusory world is real. Of necessity he must deceive them—the public, his sexual partner, and, finally, himself—in the same way that, in fantasy, he deceived the father. From there on the fear of being unmasked and punished for an unnamed crime becomes a consuming preoccupation. He must keep a close control on everything. Thus the fear of losing control is added to the anxiety of losing his fragile identity. He fears losing control, not only of himself, but also of the Other, the anonymous spectator, in whose eyes the false identity must be maintained. The image of the Other, projected onto the world of men, renders the public, all the Others, a constant threat to his position as chosen king.
>
> *(ibid., pp. 298–304)*

In this very complex and interesting passage, McDougall echoes Freud's construction of the low ego ideal in which her patient doesn't deign to enter into competition with the "siblings" or "fathers." Rather, he only has to approximate the phallic image for "the public." There are some inconsistencies between McDougall's account and mine. For example, McDougall holds that "the Oedipal situation had never been faced," but I would say that it has not been faced by the deutero part of the individual. It would be more accurate to say, following her suggestion, that the Oedipal complex was only passed through at half strength. If the paternal imago had been split by the mother, then one part of it was used to create a phallic image, and it is a part that did not experience the difference between the sexes or generations as an ego-ideal need. However, the remaining half, or part, had to experience it or there would have been no recognition of the differences between the sexes or generations, and no transcription of the phallic mother's power to the paternal. I will return to this below.

For the moment, I want to emphasize that the possession of the phallic image means that the deutero individual seems to have access to either perversions or identity quirks that play into the "narcissistic self-complacency" of the low ego ideal. McDougall's patient had a grandfather who was a writer and, strangely, McDougall does not explicitly link her patient's intellectual profession with his grandfather's. Her patient is a professor who procrastinates and only writes at the last minute. Despite this, he is still accepted as a professor, or someone who writes and produces intellectual work, by others (ibid., pp. 296, 290). McDougall does link his sadistic sexual practices to the punishment his mother had received from her own father.

McDougall's account also adds the interesting operation of "converting anxiety;" this operation, which Freud (1938b) acknowledges in his essay on splitting, observes that castration anxiety is both acknowledged in the fetish as substitute for the mother's missing phallus and disavowed by substituting the fetish for it. Along with her patient's sexual game of sadism, the procrastination is related to a social game of putting himself "into a position where [he] can't back out . . . which obliges [him] to produce" (ibid., p. 291). This relationship to anxiety, as a whole parallel economy to the economy of libido, will be examined at length in the next book.

Related to Reich's introduction of the phallic-narcissistic, and close to Jones' formulation, is Edgcumbe and Burgner's differentiation of the phallic-narcissistic and the phallic-oedipal. Regarding the former, they give the example of "a pretty, dainty, beautifully dressed child, who appeared feminine and self-satisfied . . . [and who] knew well how to make an entrance and become the center of attention, and soon became known as "the little princess" (Edgcumbe & Burgner, 1975, p. 176). Like McDougall's example, there is confidence or self-satisfaction that places the deutero phase individual above others. However, what is still lacking here is the differentiation between confidence and grandiosity, as well as entertaining different levels of this variation in self-regard in superego development. Forman (1976) builds on the phallic-narcissistic, or deutero phase, to offer a differential diagnosis of the deutero phase at phallic, anal, and oral levels (p. 55). He also importantly links this phase to the work of Kohut, but missing from his account is McDougall's more nuanced account of the phallic image, its relation to a different ego ideal, and proper references to the social body to make the differentiations.

Fairbairn (1952) similarly places the mother as the central figure in the Oedipus complex where classical analysts focused the most on the father. He writes:

> [I]t is not difficult to see that the maternal components of both the internal objects have, so to speak, a great initial advantage over the paternal components; and this, of course, applies to children of both sexes . . . In conformity with this fact, a sufficiently deep analysis of the Oedipus situation [i.e. the castration complex] invariably reveals that this situation is built up around the figures of an internal exciting mother and an internal rejecting mother . . . in the classic drama of Hamlet . . . there can be no doubt that, both in the role of exciting and tempting object and in that of rejecting object, the Queen is the real villain of the piece.
>
> *(Fairbairn, 1952, p. 124)*

Fairbairn writes that the Queen in *Hamlet* is in the role of both exciting and rejecting object, but he does not say that it is necessary that one person be in both roles. *The Lost Boys* also appears to settle on the mother as the film's central figure of power over whom the two sides fight for control. However, this does not mean that the literal mother, or a woman for that matter, are required for a phallic mother transference. The internal object aspect of the imago may retain the combined parent qualities, but the phallic mother imago (ego ideal) can be put on a man. In "Female Sexuality" (1931a) and later in his supervision of the work of

Ruth Brunswick (1940), Freud holds that the relation to the mother can be transcribed to the father. Some analysts, for example Chasseguet-Smirgel (1976a), hold that the castration complex "seems to be as proportionately intense as the maternal imago is powerful" (p. 285). In this essay, Chasseguet-Smirgel also draws attention to paternity and Athena springing from the head of Zeus. This magical form of conception without the mother shows the need to have a not-mother figure (i.e. the father) perform her functions. This also harkens back to Jones (1933) and his findings that the psychogenic denigration of women is not found in every patient and is part of the deutero phase.[14]

Freud's position on the low ego ideal and McDougall's genetic findings compel me to refine the dialectic of the relation between sexuality, ego drive, and ego ideal that I give in *The Economics of Libido* (2015). In that account, there is an id or erotic object-choice that takes the finite body of the mother as its object, and it is negated to create a not-finite, or negative sense of perfection (Freud, 1923b, pp. 29–30). The perfection, which is linked to the ego drives, in turn becomes negated, and synthesized with the mother's body, to become the *social body* through the father. Freud (1920) holds that the second step, "drive for perfection," is not based upon some innate idea of perfection, since the infinite cannot be grasped by finite minds. Instead, he sees it as an id impulse that is repressed and blocked from attaining fulfillment. It becomes a negative quality that "never ceases to strive for complete satisfaction" because "there is . . . no prospect of bringing the process to a conclusion or of being able to reach the goal" (ibid., p. 42). The sense of perfection is formulated by Freud as negative because, as it is conceived of at the phallic stage, no success in one's field of knowledge or skill can ever satisfy the person for long. A momentary triumph will always result in the perception that one can make more money, write another book, have a better batting average, etc. The social body represents the depersonalization that allows the social drives to be connected to classes/levels of authority. However, if the paternal imago is to be denigrated before the Oedipus complex, then there must be some previous link of the infinite, perfection, or not-mother negation to the father. Otherwise, how can something with a negative status be taken as an object or how can the mother's denigration of the father have any effect?

Returning to Freud's writing, I see that I missed that there is a pre-oedipal identification with the father that is found in the lead up to the Oedipus complex:

> At the same time as this identification with his father, or a little later, the boy has begun to develop a true object-cathexis towards his mother according to the attachment [anaclitic] type. He then exhibits, therefore, two psychologically distinct ties: a straightforward sexual object-cathexis towards his mother and an identification with his father which takes him as his model. The two subsist side by side for a time without any mutual influence or interference. In consequence of the irresistible advance towards a unification of mental life, they come together at last; and the normal Oedipus complex originates from their confluence.
>
> *(Freud, 1921, p. 105)*

This pre-oedipal identification suggests a sequence in which the drive for perfection that is formed at the proto-phallic phase meets with frustration. In the proto-phallic phase the mother is entreated to not just admire the body or presence of the child, as in earlier stages, but to admire the active-egoist for doing something (ex. drawing, cycling, etc.) in an *image-ego*. This something later becomes one's profession or field of work in which the egoist wants to make his mark. This drive will be frustrated, no matter how much a parent praises the child, and when it does, the infinite or perfection can be linked to the paternal, which again, for reason of pure difference, is the candidate for the not-mother. With the paternal now in place, it can either be split by the mother and used to create the deutero phase, or the paternal imago remains at full strength (i.e. creates the full ego ideal). As Freud writes in the quotation above, a new object-cathexis of the mother appears to negate the unity with the father, and this in turn is negated again to give us the ego ideal and its depersonalized relation to the social body.

A new id or erotic object-choice of the phallic mother, and not just her denigration of the father, seems important here. The mother's phallic image, as a new image of perfection for the child to try to approximate, likely comes from a mother who is "close, binding, and intimate" and stimulates the child's sexuality (Bieber et al., 1962). When we recognize that language cannot play a role in the deutero phase of early stages of development, as Forman (1976) recognizes, this non-universal adaptation must be able to rise between two bodies.

Mentioning these id object-choices brings up the important issue of the Oedipus complex as phylogenetic or ontogenetic, as mentioned above. The first has to do with the heritability of mental pathology which has statistical significance, but isn't absolute. For example, one identical twin can have schizophrenia while the other does not: therefore, what is passed on in genes is not the sole determination of pathology. The ontogenetic has to do with every child having to create the mind through the process of primary identifications that build the superego, and instinctual renunciations of id drives to form the ego drives. It must also be recognized that there are people with mental illness who do not have it in their gene pool. However, if the mind has to be ontogenetically created in each individual, how can there be an inherited plan of what does not exist? This problem is overcome by realizing that id object-choice and different expressions of aggressive impulses, for example, have an instinctual basis and do not need the ontogenetic conception of another person. The id impulses can be tied to the images of the transpersonalized imago or internal objects that are related to phantasy.

Freud (1917c, 1939) resolves the tension between the two groups of causes—nature (what is heritable) and nurture (what is created in one's own ontogenetic experience)—in his concept of the complemental series. He writes:

> [T]he gap between the two groups appears not to be unbridgeable. It is quite possible to unite the two aetiological determinants under a single conception; it is merely a question of how one defines "traumatic." If we may assume that the experience acquires its traumatic character only as a result

> of a quantitative factor—that is to say, that in every case it is an excess in demand that is responsible for an experience evoking unusual pathological reactions—then we can easily arrive at the expedient of saying that something acts as a trauma in the case of one constitution but in the case of another would have no such effect. In this way we reach the concept of a sliding "complemental series" as it is called in which two factors converge in fulfilling an aetiological requirement.
>
> *(Freud, 1939, p. 73)*

Instead of nature vs. nurture, Freud is drawing attention to the quantitative factor that leads to a trauma or the "primal repression" of the impulses, as the mediating third term (Freud, 1911b, p. 67). In other words, one can inherit a disposition to aggression or affection, along with its projection onto the internal object, at a certain stage or phase of development. However, parenting can be such that the child is not overwhelmed by it and it does not reach the necessary threshold to become a "fixation." Conversely, one's caregivers can treat one in such a way that an instinctual reaction is coaxed or born out of frustration to the point of it becoming traumatic; one can form mental pathology not part of one's gene pool. What applies to the quantitative threshold of trauma or repression, would also apply to the quantitative question of what kind of relation with the maternal imago is enough for her to become the phallic mother or a combined parent imago. Id drives of affection or sexuality, for example, may have a genetic disposition to be projected at the phallic stage so that the maternal imago is experienced as being seductive with one, even though the real caregiver might not have actively tried to denigrate the paternal imago.

III

Above I discussed Eros as fusion with the paternal imago, Phobos as the defused, ambivalent relation, and now I would like to turn to the third relation of PI or usurpation of the parental imago. In the high ego ideal, there is a binary of wanting to be viewed as competent in one's field of work that is contrasted with the PI that involves assuming the parental imago of ideal conscientiousness (i.e. one's way of working is the best or right way). In the third vignette of the first chapter, my compulsive patient described his "snarkiness" in expecting others to live up to his ideal of efficiency and good work, and this was tied to his sense of a "tyrant" and "a Hitler" who wants to "rule" over others. This was shown to be PI, and my patient originally felt this towards his own fault-finding father.

The PI with the proto paternal has definite ties with obsessive-compulsive character. As Lowen (1994) and Kurtz (2007) point out in their rigid and industrious/over-focused types, this is someone who gives the impression of being more "adult," putting too much into work life, and being prideful. The more general drive to perfection becomes transformed to perfectionism in this move, and further repression can cause specific compulsive symptoms that relate to the ego cognition of different stages of development. When other parts of the personality (i.e. following psychic bisexuality) are suppressed and the individual regresses to functioning at earlier stages, then he approaches the world in a single rigid way that is dysfunctional enough that he might come to therapy. This is when such an individual is properly held to have an obsessive-compulsive personality disorder. Otherwise, some court-mandated clients may be forced to come to therapy and present with this kind of "character armor," in PI, but I would not diagnose them with a personality disorder.

In contrast to PI with the proto paternal, Klein originally draws our attention to PI with the maternal imago, and without perfection being anchored to any ideal in work and being more responsible and "adult." She writes:

> Much of the hatred against parts of the self is now directed towards the mother. This leads to a particular form of identification which establishes the prototype of an aggressive object-relation. I suggest for these processes the term "projective identification." When projection is mainly derived from the infant's impulse to harm or to control the mother, he feels her to be a persecutor. In psychotic disorders this identification of an object with the hated parts of the self contributes to the intensity of the hatred directed against other people. As far as the ego is concerned the excessive splitting off and expelling into the outer world of parts of itself considerably weaken it. For the aggressive component of feelings and of the personality is intimately bound up in the mind with power, potency, strength, knowledge and many other desired qualities.
>
> *(Klein, 1975, p. 8)*

In Klein's formulation, if one is already perfect then the drive for perfection is not in evidence in the standard way. The synthesis with the paternal imago and the ideal of work and honor in ethical life has been lost, and power returns to the maternal imago. This means that when power is re-transcribed from the proto paternal to the proto maternal, the PI is much more debilitating and grandiose.[15] Clinically, this is borne out with low-functioning patients. For example, one patient with whom I had worked expressed how he loved the power involved in selling drugs and having people become indebted to him. He talked about the control he would have over his "minions" and how he would get them to perform crimes and do him favors. He told me that he could never last more than a day or two at a job and could not stand a boss telling him what to do. He expressed that he would always be thinking about how he could make more money in two hours than his boss could make in a week. He would sometimes make grandiose statements related to how he could "take over the world" if he just applied himself. Another patient, who was more intellectual, similarly told me about how he could cure cancer if he applied himself, but that he would not do so because people are rotten and do not deserve it.

In my job at a community clinic, I have had many low-functioning "ex-cons" make their way to mandated treatment after prison sentences. They often show little to no effort to get or keep jobs and get their lives together. They often give me the impression that they would rather remain perfect—which is an illusion that can only be kept up by not doing anything, or through always blaming others. They project all kinds of incompetence and criminality onto the legal system and exhibit a great deal of anger.[16] Their grandiosity is often adapted and more covert; it is seen through their complaining about "idiot drivers" or how others they work with have "no common sense." Such patients are very quick to express anger about the perception of weakness in others, which again follows Klein's insight into hating their own weakness from PI from usurpation of the proto maternal imago.

In summary, from the proto, to the deutero, to both parents together at the Oedipus complex, to the father complex, there is synthesis of the maternal and paternal. The mother is primary at the beginning, and is then intermingled with aspects of the father, until they are both in the forefront in the Oedipus complex. However, since the father complex phase involves the relations to siblings under the father, as possessor of the mother, it appears as if the father becomes primary at the end. This is only in regards to the internal object aspect of the imago, and as discussed, the maternal imago can be transferred to a man or vice versa in its depersonalized aspect. While the proto Oedipus complex has both parents as the imago, the non-universal deutero form has the combined parent imago, which, for the male, and following the difference between the sexes, becomes a rival male in the ego drives and a female in the object drives.

I will turn to the social functioning of the deutero phase active-egoist soon, but would first like to say a little more about the paternal proto phase. As we have seen, proto paternal figures can cause an ego injury or fixation that leads to repetition. The paternal imago represents the importance of "social anxiety" and caring about one's reputation as an ethically good person, or how one reflects on one's family, work group, or others. However, this is in combination with the earlier maternal proto phase and therefore the high ego ideal also means that the person is competitive. This creates someone who is deferential to authority because parental-substitutes receive the high ego-ideal transference, and as Freud (1931b) points out, this, along with their active-egoism, also makes them socially "conservative" (p. 218).

In contrast to the compulsive personality who is in PI with the proto paternal imago, Mackinnon and Michels (1971) discuss how traits of competitiveness and obedience show up in what they call "the obsessive patient." They see his central conflict as being between "obedience and defiance," with anger produced when he is obedient and fear produced when he engages in his indirect forms of disobedience (ibid., p. 89). In the model I am constructing, the high ego ideal means that the proto active-egoist wants to appear as competent in work and a model employee to his boss, and the parental-substitute receives a full ego-ideal transference. However, because of defusion, and a sense that one can never please the parental-substitute, that he or she never listens, or that he or she annoyingly has to be right all the time, "naughtiness" comes into play. Small acts of being late, spending too much time on a project that is not a high priority to the boss, or intentionally making little mistakes are the covert forms of disobedience. However, this is often not just one-sided. Codependency does not just show up in romantic relationships but also in dysfunctional work relationships. Often these types manage to find a parental-substitute who really is overly critical in regards to the work that the active-egoist is doing, and this attitude can sometimes be induced in the analyst or parental-substitute who normally does not feel or judge this way on their own. I would like to give an example of how this shows up clinically.

> Client is having issues with his boss. There are no overt confrontations but many small, covert ones. The boss will give client instructions for a project, but client doesn't think what he says will work. Although client carries out the instructions, he either doesn't carry them out fully or does so in a way that is designed to make them fail. Client tells me that "things aren't going the way he [his boss] envisions them working," and I ask him to do his best to describe to me how his boss might think about him at this point in their relationship. Client refers to himself as "just one of the subordinates" and says "we're stupid" and adds "you're the overlord." As he's talking his shoulders keep coming up and I ask him to close his eyes and lift them up in an exaggerated way and to tell me "what this feels like and when it reminds him of." He tries the experiment and says that it's uncomfortable and it feels like "people dealing in absolutes." and "commanding in a way of 'Because I said so . . .' without any rationale for it being that way." I ask again for him to tell me when he's felt like this before and he says with his father. He tells me that he doesn't have a specific memory, but a more general relation he's feeling towards his father. I begin BLS and ask him to stay with the relation and see what he becomes aware of.
>
> We've done this kind of work before and unprompted, he reports afterwards that he began entreating his father to work with him and told him that things didn't have to be this way. However, he reports that his father "keeps turning away" in the fantasy. I tell client that people only feel adultness when their parents foster it in them and that he'll always feel like a kid with authority figures if he lets his father turn away. We talk about why his father couldn't foster his manhood and client begins to share insight into how his father probably didn't know what he was doing as a parent and that "he wasn't the smartest man, nor the most communicative." I tell client to take these insights and to picture his father again and to tell his father that he can see his struggles, and won't let him turn away. He nods in agreement and I begin BLS. When he signals me to stop client says "that wasn't as bad as I thought it would be." I ask him for his father's response and he says, "he seemed sad and relieved," and adds, "there's something to be said when others lift burdens off of you." I ask him to picture his father looking sad and relieved and to see if his body has any reaction to this. I begin BLS and he signals that something is happening. He reports the tensions are gone and that he has a sense of calm and well-being.

I ask him to float back to another time he felt like this and he says his first promotion. I begin BLS and ask him to picture all the details he can and to let me know when they soak into him as much as they can. He goes for a bit and then signals me to stop. He says that he "feel[s] appreciated, and not used" and after some silence he adds that he "feel[s] a sense of challenge, but the challenge is something you are fully capable of mastering." He then adds that during the time of his first promotion, that he had called and asked his father's opinion about whether he should take the promotion and he remembers that his father had said "Son, I think you are fully capable: do the best you can." Client says that at the time he didn't really "need the validation," but he had called to make his father feel better, "that his son would ask his opinion . . . make him feel like he had an impact and he was part of someone else's life." Client shares the thought that his father "probably bragged" to others, and then client suddenly shares the thought that "it's sad that this is all he had" and that it should have felt like "the trophy [the promotion] is not mine, it is ours." Client adds that his father must have felt like "the odd man out" and like "he has had no impact or influence on anyone." Client tells me that he feels sad and I ask him to stay with the feeling and begin BLS. I ask him to see what his body wants. He stops and tells me "I need to give him a hug." I tell him to respect what his body wants and that he should picture his father and embrace him, but to let me know if there's another part that resists this feeling. I begin BLS and client goes for a few moments and tears stream down his face. After he signals me to stop, I ask him what his body feels like and he says, "there's a change in my core, it's mushy." I ask him if that a good or bad feeling and he laughs and has a beaming smile on his face.

This patient allows us to observe the covert defiance, the lack of a close relation to the parental-substitute, and, ultimately, the desire to want to proudly represent a leader. My patient did not have a personal relationship with his boss in or outside of work, nor did he exhibitionistically air his problems with him by putting him down in front of coworkers. Additionally, another possible connection to the Oedipus myth is found in his statements about how his triumph in the raise should have been shared with his father.[17] Oedipus became king but did not have a father with whom he could share a legacy. In contrast, in "Beyond the Pleasure Principle" (1920), Freud brings up the repetition of the benefactor abandoned in anger by each of his protégés (p. 22). I have come to see the close relation of the mentor and protégé as a special relation with authority that many people do not have, and one that is a good indication of the deutero phase. It also shows up in romantic relationships in which one party wants to change, form, or instill the "beloved" with something. I have worked with many criminals who often have children by several different women but despite these "red flags," they sometimes still have successful girlfriends who try to instill them with virtue. These women often put down the other women these men have been with, and let the men know that they will not fall for "the bullshit" that the other women did. Many encourage the men to be more successful or try to get them to go to university. The mentor/protégé relationship can also have variations like having a trusted advisor or a close friend. It is important to understand that the mentor has assumed the place of the phallic maternal imago and is projecting his self imago into his protégé so that the other completes the repetition of betrayal the mentor experienced himself (i.e. PI). Of course, it is also possible that only one party has the deutero phase or that mentor and protégé relations are part of institutional or cultural practices. It is important to examine the relation, the past relations of both parties, their character traits, etc., before determining that both share the deutero phase.

As mentioned above, by the time of the phallic stage, the active-egoist can have a relation of anaclitic love in his romantic life, but it is important to see that this can also show up with his boss. In the deutero phase, a relation of overt criticism and exhibitionistic defiance is possible with the bad phallic mother imago, or if the authority figure comes to be seen as denigrated. I will have more to say about this shortly. However, if the deutero active-egoist accepts the authority or love figure as a mentor, then there is a danger the boss or beloved can use him or take him for granted. Let me give a clinical example of this:

> Client gets into how he's going to have to quit his job, and brings up the two leads he's got for a new job. He then gets into how it's hard to leave his current job because he's "super tight with [his] boss' whole family:" client takes care of his dogs sometimes, and is "super loyal." He then gets into how his boss and his family are good people, but that they don't know how to run a business. Client tells me that there are inspectors coming by the job site and how his boss hasn't updated to the standards of the new codes. Client then explains a legitimate worry that this would affect his licenses and employability. After this he tells me how his boss had previously "made promises" regarding raises, benefits, and other things that he hasn't followed through with. Despite his boss having told "lots of lies," client still sees him as a good guy and "wants to leave on a good note." I tell client that it's hard for me to separate his boss as a person from his boss as an employer. I tell him that if I did, that it sounds like he's a shrewd business owner who is making money from cutting corners for as long as possible, and paying others as little as he can, and that he sounds like a conniving person. Client becomes reflective over this, and says that he can see my point. I ask client how his boss has been with other coworkers and he tells me that he's "fucked over others" and gets into how he did so with "the best hand we had." He also talks about another coworker with whom his boss was pretty friendly, and how this coworker quit for a better job. Client tells me that his boss "made business personal" and stopped being friends with him and made his wife stop talking to the coworker's wife. I ask client if he thinks that he might suffer the same fate as him and client is unsure but raises the feeling that it's a possibility.

I ask client to begin to describe how his boss might see him, first in a positive way and then a negative. Regarding the former, client says that his boss would think he is "a team player, talented, and that [client] will cut corners when I need him to." I ask client to say more about the last part, and it seems like besides stalling on upgrading some things to code, client's boss has actively got him to break many other codes in order to save money. I then get client to think about what his boss might think about client when he has promised him a raise but isn't giving it to him. He says that his boss thinks, "I can use him, I take him for granted," and client then tells me how his boss "caters to the workers who bitch and stand up to him." These other workers get the raises, even though they don't go "the extra mile" that client does. I ask client to continue guessing the thoughts that his boss might have about him and he adds, "he is blind, oblivious to the bigger picture." I ask client what comes to mind when he thinks of a person who is used by others and is blind and client says that such a person is "weak." I ask client to say these out as object statements, "You use me, you take me for granted, you think I'm blind, you think I'm weak." Client associates to his mother when he was a teen.

Client brings up how she convinced him to put his first car in her name to save on plates, registration, etc. and she took it from him and drove it for the next few years. He shows a little anger when he says that she "punked [him]." He brings up another time that his mother forged his signature on something and other times "she took advantage of [him]." He then adds, "you want to trust your mother," seemingly in defense of how many times he fell for this behavior. He brings up how she still expects help now and will "tag stuff on Facebook and [he] get[s] it for her and give[s] in." He then swings back to the past and talks about how she'd pick who he dated. He tells me about one girl who his mother told him that she hated, but after they split up, client says his mother and her became "best buddies" and would go to the bar together without him. We discuss this and I say that it sounds like client finds something good, a car, a girl, whatever . . . and that she takes it, or tries to. Client agrees that this feels right and then tells me that his mother "fucked one of his friends," which I can tell he feels a little embarrassed to say. I ask him for the details and he tells me that his friend was a "smooth talker" but "has never done anything productive with his life." I ask him if he was a close friend and he tells me that they were close enough but he wasn't "the kind of guy you'd introduce to your sister." He tells me that this "friend" is the kind of guy that "loves prison . . . he is all about it, he robs people," but that his [client's] mom "loved him." He strangely brings up how his mother holds a job now, as if she was the one non-productive one he had been talking about, and so I ask what she was like back when he was a teen. Client tells me that she "feared being on her own" and attached herself to men, and wasn't working, but that she got more independent after his dad left her.

> We get into the double relation he feels towards her as her "cash cow" or "golden goose" and how he feels like the "black sheep." Regarding the latter, he talks about how his mother "bitches at [him] while [he's] over there [at her place] taking out her trash." He says that she includes him in her complaints about his brothers and will say "you guys!" even though he's "not a bum like the rest of his brothers" and is the only one who actually helps her. He says that she's a "hateful, hateful human being." Regarding the former relation, client says that he's "easy to take advantage of" and that his mother can "force him to do whatever." He adds that "she's [his] mother, she gave birth to [him], and [he] kinds feel[s] like [he] owe[s] her." I ask him if he's felt this way about anyone else and he adds that he'd "do anything for his dad too, anything for family."

The ego and object statements in this vignette show that the deutero, close relationship to the boss is a repetition of what my patient experienced with his mother. His language at the end also shows that the phallic stage brings the active individual to not only full love with a romantic object, but that this can also be expressed regarding a boss and belonging to a family. Although my patient described himself as a "team player," and sees this as a strength, his specialness or exceptionality is seen in how he did not want to be lumped in with his brothers and he how does more than them. This clinical example sets up how the active individual can be "robbed" in his loyalty to the phallic mother, but also has material concerning the reverse. My patient's "smooth-talking friend" who "has never done anything productive with his life" shows the opposite attitude of seeking to rob others.[18] With some active patients, this robbing can be projected on the opposite sex, so that a girlfriend might be described in object statements as "she is a gold digger, she does nothing for herself, she just wants someone to support her, she loves money." These statements can be turned into ego statements, when there is enough rapport. The active patient can admit that they feel true for him, and that in his previous way of living, he was looking for "a free ride" and saw others as "dumb, worthless, and naïve," and he would "steal from you, and take everything you had."[19]

The Lost Boys presents variations of these deutero dynamics. Although we are not given a close, mentor- and protégé-like relationship, David has a special interest in Michael that is the foundation for such a relationship. Additionally, Michael defeats David at the end and there is a sense of rough equality between them, although Michael is only a half-vampire and much more inexperienced with his powers. This follows the low ego-ideal sense of the parental-substitute receiving less idealization while the ego increases in self-regard. As mentioned in the last chapter, there are moments in which David appears much more powerful, but also moments in which Michael is represented as his peer, but with David having an edge, such as with his "throbbing," superior motorcycle. Additionally, the binary of robbing or being robbed is important and strongly visible in *The Lost Boys*. The lost boys live outside of society and come in to rob others of their blood or life, and Sam steals Grandpa's car in parallel to Michael stealing Star from David. Lastly,

Michael does not accept David's special interest in him because he wants to be "his own man," in parallel to Sam wanting to remain "man of the house," but also because David is viewed as bad (as wanting to make him into a murderer). I will return to this idea of the bad phallic mother again later on, but for the moment I want to keep fleshing out the manifestations of this phase.

When there is acceptance of the phallic mother imago, in contrast to the relation of Michael and David, there is a built-in pattern of idealization and debasement. This can be understood as repeating the relationship in which the phallic mother, whose power has been transcribed to the paternal, becomes debased. After creating the phallic image in the child, she becomes "castrated" and no longer has the phallus. In the clinical example of the double in Chapter 2, the idealization and then debasement was explicitly stated, and my patient ended up in the place of the "castrated" phallic mother whose "world is on fire." In the session, he questioned God along the following lines, "I don't understand . . . you made me so special, how come I don't get a family, a wife, and those things . . . how come I don't get those things?" "How come I'm so different than other people?" He was able to reverse this PI and within the fantasy he put the ex-girlfriend's world on fire, thus transforming from the position of "the zero." In many active deutero patients, what is common is the idea of the romantic object, mentor, advisor, or friend who is stringing one along. They are either "riding one's coat tails," treating one as a golden goose, or they can be "frustrating" by withholding knowledge, secrets, full intimacy, or the complete phallic image for the active-egoist.

The primal scene, as a specific repetition, involves betrayal from the mentor, advisor, or romantic partner, or seeing the phallic mother (substitute) being traumatically attacked. This stands in contrast to the regular idealization and debasement cycle. In working with many poor, chemically dependent patients, I have been amazed to see how powerfully repetition governs people's lives. There are men and women who have been cheated on in nearly every relationship they have been in, with this sometimes including the additional ego injury of being cuckolded by a close friend more than once.[20] In the realm of the ego drives, pursuing one's career or being proud of some skill or knowledge in a field of interest can leave one similarly open to being humiliated by someone who attempts to unmask one as grossly incompetent or inferior. Again, the person who is doing the humiliating, if it is a pattern for him, is doing so in PI. A man can go around cuckolding other men, but he can also go around trying to embarrass others in their professions as chef Gordon Ramsay, for example, has made a career out of.

When the primal scene involves witnessing the phallic mother being disrespected, injured, or humiliated, this is akin to her castration. Clinically, many people take on the place of the castrated phallic mother in a way that will keep the therapy stuck if it is not undone. Many of the criminal patients I see are on probation, and they can be fixated on the unfairness of having to "jump through hoops," often complaining that the police are not so innocent themselves. They have fantasies of reversing the positions they are in and want the police, or their probation officers, to feel what it is like to be as "controlled" or dominated as they feel. They imagine that these officers enjoy putting them "down" or having them "beneath" them. I would like to give two clinical examples and then talk about the common structure in such cases:

> Client obsessively talks about the DA and whether the court system will send him to prison or not. It's one thing to worry about the future when other people have control, but it's another to talk about the figures involved in an overly personal way when one doesn't know them. I try to get into some assertiveness work with him and away from the topic of the DA. He either lets people walk all over him, or a dissociated part of his personality makes him feel like someone is making him out to be a "bitch" or "punk" and he wants to fight. He's pushed away the exploration of his passive side before and because he had other issues that needed to be attended to, I allowed it. Recently I began stressing that this passive side needs to learn to stand up for itself, because the dissociated identity has come out and threatened some people. He gives some recent examples of his passivity with some renters who have not paid him rent for several months. I ask him why it's important that someone pays him rent and he gives me good practical reasons. I ask him to picture one of the renters and to tell him those reasons but, after I begin BLS, he isn't even able to confront him in his own imagination. He says that the idea of "cutting someone off who is really trying" bothers him too much. I ask him if anyone has ever done that to him and he says the DA (referring to how he is awaiting sentencing for a recent conviction). I ask him to focus on this, begin BLS, and he gets in touch with tensions in his stomach. The BLS continues and he says that he feels like he could get sick. I ask him to vomit in his mind's eye and give into what his body wants. During the BLS, I ask him to picture who shows up on the receiving end of it (i.e. who he'd like to vomit on). He signals that the scene has played out and tells me that the DA showed up and that the tensions and nausea left him. However, he reports that he now feels tired.
>
> I ask him to stay with this tired feeling and to see what it wants (i.e. for him to collapse, for him to leave his body, or other common responses). He says that he doesn't feel like he wants to collapse, but instead says that a picture of a rock hammer, "worn down to the nub" appeared in his mind. He associates this to *The Shawshank Redemption* (1994) and I ask him for his first thoughts about this movie. He says that the main character is tenacious and was in a bad situation and prevailed. I have heard him talk about this part of himself before, but I want him to stay with the tired part of himself that he just got in touch with, so I don't explore this association. I ask him to describe the image of the rock hammer and he says it is "beat up, fucked up, and used up." I ask him if it feels true if he says these things about himself. He says it does and gets in touch with a "hollow" feeling in his chest. I resume BLS and he feels it grow, but then it doesn't lead to anything. I ask him to project it out and tell me what someone or something would

look like if he, she, or it looked like he felt. He says, "humpty dumpty" and quickly adds, "an empty egg." I ask him to picture Humpty Dumpty and then the environment he imagines him in. He follows the traditional story that Humpty Dumpty is on a wall, falls, breaks, and is put back together and in the end he pictures him as "cracked all over" and "not whole." I ask client to picture the cracked egg that is made up of pieces in his chest and to see if it feels right there. He affirms that he can map it onto his sensations there, and then complains that a sharp pain has appeared in his lower back. I continue with the BLS, but the pain continues to grow instead of diminishing. Client compares the pain to being "twisted" in his pelvis and lower back and I ask him to imagine that someone is twisting him and causing this pain to him. He says "it's the legal system." I ask him if anyone specific comes to mind and he says the DA.

I ask him to imagine that the DA is the one who is literally twisting him and to just pay attention to his body's reaction to this scene in his head. I begin BLS and after some moments he signals me to stop and reports that it feels like he's "losing energy" and "giving in" instead of feeling any anger or fight in him. Based upon work with many others who have had this response and who on their own had imagined that someone else begins to appear in the scene, I introduce a third person myself. I ask my patient to imagine that a "random, neutral person walks in on what the DA is doing to him" and to tell me what he or she would think about the situation. He says that the person would think that "it's bullshit" and that "the giant picks on the little guy . . . like David and Goliath." I ask him what the person would say to him or the DA, and he says, "leave him alone," "you're an asshole." I then ask him what the person would think of him in this scene and he says that "he would see I'm in extreme pain." I get him to put these into object statements, as if he was the random person (i.e. "This is bullshit, you are an asshole, you're in extreme pain, etc."). He says that when he was a kid that he'd watch his stepfather beat his mother when he was drinking and client details the times that come to mind. I begin BLS and he gets in touch with wanting to protect his mother and being scared because he is so small. I tell him to stay with both the feeling of wanting to protect her and being afraid and to see which one is stronger. He says wanting to protect her, but he also adds that he feels like he can't do anything. I tell him to imagine that he goes into the memory as he is now (i.e. his current adult self) and to see if it feels different. After BLS, he tells me that he tackled his stepfather. I ask him to scan his body and see if more needs to come out. He says that he lost his anger and that sadness has come up. He talks about how his stepfather was only bad like this when he drank and that he only wanted to restrain him to let his mother go. I ask him to stay with the sadness and he gets into how it was wrong for his kid self to have had to see this. He also brings up what it must have been like for his siblings to see this too and I affirm that he's right and that no kid should have to see this. I ask him to picture his stepfather sober with his mother, to tell them what he just told me, and begin BLS. He signals me to stop and tells me that he told them and that they look ashamed and own up to it, and know it's wrong. He begins to cry and I tell him that this is the hurt kid in him and that he needs to let it move through him. He continues to cry and when he finishes I ask him to picture his parents again. He says that they look sad and remorseful. I ask him to keep picturing this reaction in them and to see how his body reacts to seeing this. He says that he begins to feel warm and that he feels warm all throughout his chest (where he was formerly hollow). I ask him to remember a time that he felt like this, and he said it's recent, it's when his mother told him that she was proud of him. I ask him to picture her face and hear her words, and to let me know when he feels that they have come into him as much as they can. I begin BLS. He tells me that the warmth spreads even further.

Another patient is struggling with both his probation officer and a girlfriend who he doesn't trust. He can drive himself to despair with the idea that his girlfriend might be cheating with another man. He can feel anger towards the interloper in this scenario, and wants to "break his jaw," but he can't access any anger towards her. When he isn't focused on the other man, he rails against probation. He bitterly tells me that they should be chasing sex offenders and serious criminals and not wasting time with him for nothing. My patient had committed more serious crimes, but got in trouble for smoking cannabis while on probation. He gets uncharacteristically poetic and compares himself to a "little balloon that's floating" and his probation officer (PO) (and the legal system in general) is "yanking him by his string" and "jerking" him around. Words like "ridiculous, retarded, and dumb" are constantly used as I encourage him to vent. He adds, "how would they like it if they were one of us and had to follow the rules like us." He begins to calm down and adds, "I feel like I got robbed." With his anger beginning to die down I ask him to tell me what kind of person robs someone else, and to tell me any words that feel right to describe these people. He says they have a "hard-nosed, prickish attitude," and adds, "they piss me off." I ask him to use these as ego and object statements and he says his best friend, who he caught in bed with an ex-girlfriend, his mom, and his foster parents come up. I ask him to focus on his best friend and his ex, but he just ignores me and continues to complain about his PO. I meet him where he's at and ask how the PO might see him? Client says that he is seen as "just a number, a ward of the state, a nobody, and not important." I ask him what the PO wants to do to him, and he says that his PO thinks, "I'm going to overpower you, to punish you."

I ask client to focus on this relation and begin BLS. He suddenly feels a pain in his shoulder and as I continue BLS it doesn't go away. I ask client to stay with the pain and imagine that someone is beside him, causing this pain to him, and he should tell me the first person he imagines is doing it. He says

> it is his PO. I ask him to picture him and to see if his body has a reaction to it. He doesn't feel any reactive anger, but feels like he's weak and giving in. I ask him to imagine that a random, neutral person shows up to see this and what this person might think about his attacker. He says, "you're a lunatic, you're crazy, you're angry." I ask him what this person thinks of him and he says, "you're a victim, weak, helpless." He imagines that the neutral stranger says, "Stop that! You're hurting him." I ask Client to imagine he's in the place of the stranger and to say these statements about two people from his past. He tells me that a "buddy" of his was shot in a home invasion by a rival gang and was killed. I ask him to stay with this memory and begin BLS. He reports that it's too disturbing and I ask him to re-present the scene to himself and imagine he is looking at it through a keyhole in my office door. He agrees, I begin BLS, and he reports that it's not as strong this way. We proceed to desensitize the memory and he discharges the fear and emotions and processes it.

Although the primal scene is often represented as involving a betrayal of parental love, Freud also registers that it shows up in ego-drive relationships. For example, in the case of the Wolfman, Freud (1918) emphasizes the sexual aspects of the Wolfman's mother as submissive and dominated by the father, but he adds that "in *this case* the significance was limited to the sexual sphere" (p. 41, *emphasis added*). He also writes of the Wolfman's submissiveness in the social sphere: "In the later years of his childhood each of his tutors and masters played the part of his father, and was endowed with his father's influence both for good and for evil" (ibid., p. 39). With my second patient, we can see that it need not involve the actual mother, but whoever receives the phallic mother transference: in this case his friend. In other words, what is important is not an episode of trauma during psychosexual development, but that the imago relations formed there can be defused and/or are open to ego injuries/trauma later, after psychosexual development. This patient got over his fixation after clearing out the emotions from witnessing his friend get attacked. No earlier episode with his parents emerged in the work for the fixation to be resolved. My first patient had the father-substitute of the DA and was in the place of his mother, who he saw his stepfather beating up. Socially, both patients felt trapped and in the possession of the DA or PO who gets to hurt him and dominate him with impunity.

I have four more notes to make about the deutero relation. First, in the cases in which the deutero phase is created by a seductive phallic mother, this aspect of the relationship is often transcribed to the father in the ego drives for the male. Connecting this idea to *The Lost Boys*, one cannot help but feel that the relation of Michael and David is a little homo-erotic.[21] Second, Freud contrasts the devil with God as potential father-substitutes in 'A Seventeenth-Century Demonological Neurosis' (1923a). Fairbairn (1952) takes up the case of Christoph that Freud discusses here to emphasize the necessity of an imago relation, so that a person will choose an evil or bad imago rather than be without one. He writes:

> [F]or the whole point of a pact with the Devil lies in the fact that it involves a relationship with a bad object . . . he sold his eternal soul to obtain, accordingly, was not gratification, but a father, albeit one who had been a bad object to him in his childhood.
>
> *(Fairbairn, 1952, pp. 71–72)*

Again, in *The Lost Boys*, David appears as a bad phallic mother-substitute with a special interest in Michael. Michael has to try very hard to resist killing, so as to not become a full-vampire, and become bad himself. It is important to consider that there are still hierarchies and relationships to authority among people who steal from and murder others (i.e. organized crime) and these groups illustrate fusion with a bad imago. Examples of going against the dominant religion and choosing the devil, or going against the laws and joining a gang, are very overt, but examples of joining subcultures, using vulgar language, and other more covert forms are also seen in the clinic. The issue of whether these manifestations are part of socialization and ego identifications with dominant people in one's life, or part of individual superego relations, has to be determined in each individual case. Fairbairn does not supply many clinical examples so it is difficult to know how he is using the good and bad binary. For my purposes here, I hold the bad imago to be one with which the individual does not want to enter into relations, and as one that the individual feels will taint him morally if he does get close to it. The good imago is the one with which one gets into close relations, but it can still be frustrating, rejecting, and cause ego injuries.

Following the difference between a good but frustrating phallic mother and a bad one, a common clinical phenomenon I see in working with chemical dependence is how a patient becomes his bad father. While some patients can describe their father in negative ways, they had very much behaved in similar ways themselves. During treatment, I can often use the same adjectives that they used to describe their father as ego statements about themselves and they will tell me that they feel true for (a part of) them. As the phenomenon developed, I began to notice that many had not even met their fathers and that the negative traits were what they had been told by their mothers. The patient becoming like their bad father was a direct reference to "becoming what their mother hated most." Again, asking them if it feels true to say this about themselves was answered in the affirmative and could often be linked to reacting to the negative traits of their mothers (i.e. "she's controlling," "she complains and is never happy," "she thinks she is perfect and never admits to mistakes," "if I stayed with her to take care of her I'd have no life," etc.).

One of the striking things about the myth of Oedipus is that he blinds himself after finding out that he married his own mother. Since Tiresias, the seer, is represented as having breasts and being a combined parent imago, and is also blind, it is possible that the blindness of Oedipus might symbolize how he becomes Tiresias. However, it seems more likely to me that Tiresias represents a combined parent imago that is related to the proto paternal and not the phallic mother of the deutero phase. Regardless, I would like to offer a clinical example of this insight:

Client is a natural leader. In groups, he can give good advice and others respond well to him. He confidently asserts himself with women as well and people seem taken by his confidence. In individual session, he shares a dream that he goes to jail to see his ex-girlfriend's new boyfriend. He says that he meets with him in a visiting room, and that the boyfriend is wearing plain clothes that are "super dark navy blue." Client says they have a talk about a disagreement concerning his son and that he feels like it goes well. The dream fragment has a positive feeling overall. Client associates first to the waiting room. He says that it reminds him of seeing his brother who is serving a significant sentence in prison. He talks about finding out that his brother listened to him and "cliqued up" with a gang in prison for protection. Client says that he set him up with "a good group of dudes" and smiles at me in a self-satisfied way. Client generally feels like his brother "looks up to [him]" and like he "did right by him" and spent time with him in order to put him on the "right path." Client seems to be bragging in letting me know his connections with prison gangs and that he had enough pull to set up his brother, but I do not have strong counter-transference with which to work.

I ask client to associate navy blue and "cops" is his first association. I ask him for his first thought about the police and he says that he "hates them" and that it feels like "they always try to control [him]." I ask for examples and he gives a time when he was a kid and his mother called one over to the house who had threatened to "beat him up." Client then talks about the police trying to catch him when he was out past curfew when he got a little older. I point out that cops are authority figures and ask him about how he feels about bosses, teachers, counselors, etc. He says that he struggles with every authority figure and feels like "no one has his best interest at heart" and that he ends up "fighting everything." He brings up how when dealing with certain people he even catches himself "twisting information to suit himself best." He tells me that he has to stop himself from trying to manipulate me, but adds that I'm not like other counselors. I ask him the first thing that comes to mind when he thinks about really trusting someone and he says, "laying down and taking shit." He quickly adds, "I feel like I'm the only one who fights for me," and tries to change the subject and get away from the idea of surrender. I've built up some credit with him over a few sessions and so I push and ask him to stay with the feeling of laying down and taking shit and begin BLS. He tells me that he sees "glimmers" of courtrooms and interactions with a cousin and feeling "helplessness." As he's talking his shoulders keep raising. I ask him to exaggerate the movement and hold them up and to close his eyes and tell me "what it feels like and when it reminded him of?" He tells me that he feels nauseous and says that women flash before his eyes: ex-girlfriends and his mother. He begins to feel anger and tells me that "women think they are always right, even when they are wrong." I ask him to stay with the feeling and to tell me who sticks out the most as always being right and begin BLS. He says his mother comes up strongest and then he tells me stories about how she tries to "control" his brothers and that they go to her for help and money and how he escaped her control. I ask him to compare this feeling with the feeling he has with the police. He shows a flash of insight and says that they are the same.

Based on material from a previous session, I venture an interpretation with the dream. I tell him that that his girlfriend's new boyfriend is there as a cover and that he is really a police officer and that there is a part of him that wants to go back to jail. Based upon client talking about his father being in and out of prison for drug use and his mother's distaste for him in a previous session, I interpret that he "looks up to" his father as a way to escape his mother's control. I say that just as he feels that he's his brother's role model, that his father is his and that he's become the thing that his mother hates, his father. Client again shows a flash of insight and reports that he feels tightness in his chest. I begin BLS and he says his heart feels "wrinkly and squished" and compares the feeling to a sponge. I continue BLS and he reports that he's starting to feel "empty and sleepy." I ask him to give in to it and continue BLS. The feeling deepens and he notes more weakness. I tell him to stay with it and ask him if it feels like he wants to collapse. He nods in the affirmative and I continue BLS. He then stops following my fingers and shares that he saw a picture of a woman, who is "super blond," but who is a "sketch" or "stick figure." I ask him to see if he can internalize this image and see if it feels right to picture it in his chest and resume BLS. He says that it feels right but that he can only partly map it on to the sensations there. I see him wince and he tells me that he doesn't want it to come in. Our time is up and I don't have time to explore what in him rejects it. I just end the session.

In the next session, we get to a point in which client is talking about an ex and how her parents "threw him for a loop" by making up lies about him at court. He said he "didn't expect it" and puts most of the blame on the mother who he says is "a bitch" and then tells me that he "hates her." While talking about the father, who he thinks is "respectable," he narrows his left eye and adds, "I didn't respect him totally." I mimic how his left eye narrows and ask him to recreate this face, hold it, and tell me how it feels. He does so and says it reminds him of how he feels when he "gets in trouble with the law and has to suffer the consequences." I ask him for some times that come to mind and begin BLS, but he says that it's barely showing up. I ask him if he had any other times or thoughts about closing his eye and he tells me that it reminds him of the sun. I ask him to describe his general thoughts about the sun. He tells me that he "like[s] it" but sometimes it can be "too bright." He continues and calls it "too hot" and adds that he has to "look away" or "turn [his] back on it." I retool these in an anthropomorphic way, and ask him to say them about someone from his past as ego and object statements: "I like you, but you are too bright. I can't be with you, you get me too hot. I have to look away or turn my back on you." Client says that "people in general" come up. He talks about a friend and how he has a pattern with people: he "like[s] them at first but then begin[s] picking them apart." He gets into how this is especially true of all the women he's been with. He talks about them as "ass" and how his friends tease him sometimes about bringing "a chick" around and how quickly she disappears and is replaced by another.

I ask client to focus on the statements about the sun and how things feel with the women he is with. He says things like "they get too wrapped up in my shit," they are "too needy," that he doesn't "have a lot of time" and "they are nosy." I ask him to talk about how they might think about him: from how things were at first, to when he started to feel like he wanted to "turn his back on them." He says that they'd say, "you used to be around more, you were more into me, you used to put in more time and effort, and were more attentive." I ask him to take these statements and say them about someone else and see who they feel right with. He tells me that an ex comes up, one of the two women he says that he's really loved or cared for, and he feels tension in his stomach. I begin BLS. He says that the sensation isn't very strong and I ask him to refocus on how his ex used to be close to him, but then wouldn't give him the same amount of time or attention and resume BLS. He says that the sensation has grown bigger and filled his whole abdomen. I ask him to see if any expression wants to come out of it and resume BLS. He says that he doesn't feel that any expression wants to come out and after I continue, he tells me that it's getting smaller. I notice that client has tears in his eyes and I point this out to him and he says he doesn't want to feel sad for her. I ask him to see if he can let the sadness come in. He says he hates her and doesn't want to. We go back and forth a little and I explain to him that if he doesn't let this feeling come in that it will come back to affect him in other ways.

Client capitulates and says he will try to let the sadness in. However, when I begin BLS again he tells me that it is "hard to find; it's hard to see it." I think of the stick figure from last session and tell him that he seems like he can't find his emotions (at least the vulnerable ones). I tell him that it makes me think of the stick figure of the blond and the expressionless quality of it. I ask him to picture it again and see if it can map into his chest. He agrees to try but then tells me that it maps on a little but "not much at all." I tell him that emotions are in bodies and not in sticks and that he should picture the stick figure and see the first woman who comes to mind that is full-bodied. He says that he pictures the sketch becoming the ex that we had just talked about. I ask him what she looks like (the expression on her face). He says she is smiling and looks happy. I ask him to try to picture this image of her and bring it into his chest and begin BLS. He puts her in and reports that she maps on. I ask him to let her fully embed in there and to then see what his body does with this image and continue BLS. He then signals for me to stop and says the tension in his chest is gone and that he feels less anxious. He says there is "calm" in

> his chest now and I ask him to focus on it and tell me another time he felt this well-being. He tells me a memory of camping with friends and I anchor it in. After this he spontaneously reports that he "feels normal" and like he did a few years back when he felt connected with people.

Although there are vignettes that more directly show how statements about the father become affirmed ego statements, I chose this vignette because it allows me to touch on a few other issues too. First, working with the body allows for the psychoanalyst to see if an interpretation causes a reaction and is a form of verification. The interpretation about becoming his father met with unconscious resistance and could not be accepted by my patient, but it was important to know for future sessions that it was right. Second, this example shows how the difference between the sexes often becomes part of pathology in the deutero phase with my patient universalizing about women and half-consciously getting revenge on them. My patient engaged in PI with the pain he got from his ex and began pseudo-relationships with women in which they idealized him but he would pull back in order to cause them to feel the rejection and abandonment that he had felt. These relationships with the women did not stop after this session. As usual, there was a confluence of several drives that chose this expression. However, he eventually was able to enter a monogamous relationship after a couple of more months.

The third point is that mentor-protégé deutero relationship has ties to what Kohut (1971) calls a mirror transference. Based upon the model I am introducing here, there is a big difference between PI with the proto-parental imago in which the self imago inferiority tensions of the ego ideal are put into others and the repetition of mentor and protégé relations in the deutero phase. Kohut does not make this differentiation, and he also holds that the grandiose self arises due to the failure of the caregivers to mirror the child in psychosexual development, as opposed to the close, binding, and intimate relation with the phallic mother. However, he also includes an "alter-ego" or "twinship" transference to be included in the egoistic/narcissistic line, which would have parallels with the phallic mother relation.[22] For example, when the mother praises the child as like her, worthy of investment with the phallic image, and different than the denigrated father, there is sameness established. Similarly, the mentor often "sees himself" in the protégé and would like to give extra time and special attention to him.

The fourth, and last point, concerns how the phallic mother's phallus can also express a romantic relationship. I have indicated that David's motorbike is represented as his phallic advantage over Michael, but in clinical work there is sometimes an equation between a man's prized possession and his wife or girlfriend. For example:

> One patient comes in with a dream that he's working on a vehicle, a van, in his garage. His deceased father comes in and he reports that he had a question for him, but can't remember what it was. The thing that stuck out to him was that his father's face kept changing back and forth with his uncle's.

> His first association to the van is that he had bought one a few years back, put a few hours into it and had sold it for more than double what he had bought for it. I ask him about the person to whom he had sold it but this specific transaction didn't register in any strong way for him, and so I asked him to talk to me about generally buying and fixing vehicles like this. His association to this was that his current car, is one that he's put a good deal of money into and he said he's "really attached" to the car. He even adds that he'd "burn it before [he'd] sell it." This is an interesting relation and so I ask him to describe the car. He says, "it looks good, and it's big." I ask him to say this about someone else and to tell me if anyone comes to mind (i.e. you look good, you are big, I'd rather burn you (destroy you) than lose you." He says that his wife comes up and then adds that he "couldn't stand to see her with anyone else" and adds that he'd "have to move." I ask him to stay with this idea of losing her and begin BLS. He reports he feels it strongly in his chest and I ask him to stay with the feeling and then tell me other times in his past in which he felt like this.

Culturally, we can recognize this kind of relation in the idea of trophy wives. The wife is part of the vanity of a rich man and is not chosen for love. She is just another "prized possession" and is a phallic sign, as opposed to symbol, for such a man's status. A phallic symbol, as mentioned in Chapter 1, is literally something shaped like a penis, and can be associated to it, by its physical form. A sign, in contrast, need not refer to the physical form and a woman, a watch, a car, and other things that often don't have a penis-like shape are examples. In the literature, Fenichel (1949) appears to be the first analyst to have made this connection.

Returning to *The Lost Boys*, this aspect of the deutero phase raises the question of whether Star, along with his superior motorbike, is a phallic sign of David? As we will see in the next data analysis, there is a strong connection to Michael stealing Star from David's vampire lair as a rationalization for Sam stealing Grandpa's prized car. However, even if this is the case, this does not preclude that Michael also has a proto paternal, idealizing love towards Star. Granted, it will be diminished in strength, because the paternal imago has been split in half, but David's blood connection to Star definitely references her as familial and proto paternal.

We have seen that Michael's two main relations to David are stealing Star away from him and resisting his band of lost boys (and becoming a full vampire). We have seen how Sam ruins Lucy's dates with Max by invoking Michael (and vampires) and thus steals Lucy from him, and escapes Max's authority in the latent plot. In this regard, Lucy appears as the phallic sign for who will be "man of the house." Moreover, although Sam gets into bed with Lucy, she is portrayed as morally good and instead of Sam literally being in love with her, their relationship is probably best understood as Lucy being a repersonalized imago for him. Additionally, Max also figures as the remaining half of the paternal imago (i.e. the difference between the generations and the suitable adult partner that Lucy should have). He is not just the bad phallic mother who wants to take Sam's authority or freedom to be "his own man," and Sam senses him to have a connection to Lucy, just as David has a blood connection to Star. Although both phases are discernable, it is clear that dynamically, the deutero phase is much more prominent than the proto paternal. In the next data analysis, I will go further with the deutero phase and explore the denigrated paternal imago, the phallic image, and more in the film.

Notes

1 At times Freud still oscillates with contrasting the ego drives with the sexual drives, or the object drives with the self-preservative drives, or object libido with narcissistic libido, in his work.

2 I am very much open to the argument that these cases are simply a displacement from humans to animals, and that sublimation requires a reference to such drives in combination with a commitment to one's profession or field of work, or involves a reference to bodily zones and/or their related materials. Sorting through the widely divergent literature on this subject is outside of my interest here.

3 "We call this organization their 'ego.' Now there is nothing new in this. Each one of us makes this assumption without being a philosopher . . . In psycho-analysis we like to keep in contact with the popular mode of thinking and prefer to make its concepts scientifically serviceable rather than reject them" (Freud, 1926b, p. 195).

4 Freud's formulation of the elation in mania is another example of becoming one's own ego ideal or assuming the parental imago (Freud, 1917d, pp. 253–255; 1921, pp. 131–133).

5 Talking about conscientiousness about one's chosen field of work will strike some readers as naïve, since there are surely people who get into positions of status or power who have little talent and have relied on charisma, manipulation/deception, or criminal activities to get them there. The reason I am pointing to ego drives that concern work life is to follow one trend in some people's personalities and show how deep it can go. However, this is obviously not very important in *The Lost Boys*, and I will get into how Freud conceptualizes those for whom work is not important later on in the discussion.

6 Freud contrasts the active-egoistic and the passive-altruistic ego drives and the latter will be explored in the next book. For the moment, I'll just compare the common language usage of egoism to the ego drives that aim at "perfection," "magnification of the individual," "mastery," and that Freud also compares to Adler's "will to power" (Freud, 1917a, p. 137; 1924, p. 163; 1933, p. 96). Freud often reverts to his earlier formulation of the drives of self-preservation, even in his late phase, but instead of a banal connection to hunger, or other basic functions, I'd ask my reader to consider that the different estimates of parental power by which one measures oneself, give the sense of self-preservation across both bodily need, as well as different social levels.

7 As seen in the fourth clinical example in Chapter 1, shame/remorse can cause an ego injury that leads to repetitions (with possible PI).

8 Of course, this game of honor in the ethical life of the community mediates one's relation to the stranger or non-intimate. When it comes to intimates who have the ego ideal put on them, feelings like loyalty are tied to a trans-historical morality and become important in symptom formation (Freud, 1921, p. 106).

9 I hope that I do not have to write that women can also have the ability to make, and gain self-respect from, promises too. However, not all men or women finish psychosexual development with this ability, nor with dominant character on their active-egoistic pole.

10 The term "narcissistic" is over-used in psychoanalysis and perhaps it might be better to contrast the neurotic individual to the sociopath, for example.

11 This difference can be defended against, but object-drive defenses that remain heterosexual are not necessarily superior to homosexual ones. A heterosexual can be unable to love or may repeat relationships in which the "beloved" is abandoned or hurt, while a homosexual relationship can show real affection, vulnerability, and commitment. Freud

also gives evidence for both defensive causes of homosexual desire as well as non-defensive causes, but this is too complicated an issue to investigate here.

12 There are many examples of these types of aggression: biting, spitting, sliming, beheading, dismembering, castrating, blinding, etc. However, Freud (1933) also indicates that id forms of affection are present and are similarly related to anxiety (p. 120). Just as children's books and cartoons can feature monsters and strong heroes, they can also be about cute, cuddly, and caring figures.

13 I was surprised in my clinical experience that the phallic mother shows up so easily with some patients. Some people can report dreams in which there is a literal woman with a penis. I have also had some patients who have dreams of men with breasts. These combined parent imagos sometimes represent power but also humiliation and being castrated. I would like to provide a brief vignette on how this can also show up in covert, symbolic form:

> Client brings up problems with his girlfriend defensively. Whenever he engages in progressive communication and offers up a new facet of his life, he can tangentially bring up his girlfriend. Almost every time it is to display how much he loves her, is devoted to her, and if she'd only love him back, then his life would be happy. In one session, he reveals that his mother put him in foster care and begins to tell me that he's "weak," that I "have no idea about how weak [he is]," and he's "got no backbone." Then, tangentially, he says that he gave his girlfriend a few hundred dollars and "didn't even ask any questions about it" because he "want[s] her to be happy." He emphasizes that he didn't ask her how she spent it, which is a big deal to him because he constantly questions whether she is cheating on him. Several times he references that she has "the key to his heart" and that "she's better than she's acting." I ask for his association to key and he says skeleton key. I ask him to picture a skeleton key and to think about where it would be used. He says the county jail. I ask him to imagine that he's in the jail and to imagine who has the key or where it is there. He imagines a female guard who has the key and "strolls like a bitch" and "taunts the prisoners." She acts like, "I got you . . . bye bitches" as she walks past. I ask him how he and the other inmates react to this and he says that the other prisoners reach out to get her through the cell bars, but no one can reach her. He adds the strange idea that as they reach for her their hands fall off, and that they just have "little nubs" at the end of their arms. I ask him to imagine that he has little nubs at the end of his arms and begin BLS. He says it feels right to imagine them there and that he feels "powerless and frozen" and has the feeling "fuck I'm here again."

14 Of course culture might pass on ideas of women's inferiority to people. The difference is whether analysis will show certain psychological defenses or bad representations of imagos vs. whether the person has merely submitted to the authority of popular opinion or expectations without the imagos showing an inner need to see women that way.

15 I use the term re-transcribed in homage to Bergler (1938) who uses "transcription" to designate "executive power from mother to father" and "renewed transcription" for the reversal (p. 518). Lacan's term of foreclosure comes close to this operation but he links it directly to psychosis/delusion (Lacan, 1993, 2007). However, psychosis/delusion is not always an issue for patients who have reversed transcription and Bergler is closer to the operation I see here. In my experience re-transcription is important for borderline patients, and psychosis is a defense that requires something more than the return of power to the maternal.

16 Clinically, some borderline and psychotic patients have put forward material in which their mother or women in general are attributed with terrible perfection and malice (i.e. with disregard for regular ethical life). The re-transcription of power from the paternal imago to the proto-maternal imago may be a key factor in borderline patients who often show severe self-criticism that is commensurate with the high ego ideal.

17 With several active-egoistic patients, in which the focus of them performing well in their field comes up, there is not just an issue with disobedience. Sometimes there is an ego injury from the feeling of having disappointed the parent or parental-substitute.

One patient had been trained by his father in martial arts. He made it to the city championship fight but lost the fight. He admitted that he had "a hard time with losing" and would throw things or walk off by himself and want to be alone after he lost (not just in martial arts but other sports too). In getting to this memory of the city championship he expresses that the feeling "kinda sucks" and that he had probably been "a poor sport." He then expresses that he might have got "too big of a head" because he had won many matches before and had built up a good reputation and was "a bit of a legend already." He then tells me about the car ride home from the tournament and how he felt like he let his father down and there was a "strong silence" in the car that imparted a strong sense of having disappointed him. He gets further into the feeling and wishes that he would have apologized to him. I ask him to go into his mind's eye and to apologize and say whatever else needs to come out, until he feels like he's discharged this feeling. After BLS, he reports that the feeling is gone and that he has the sense that his father accepted his apology and he tells me that he feels "at peace with it."

18 This binary does not register as my patient being in PI with the phallic mother imago since he explicitly references being part of his boss' company and his mother's family. Instead, it concerns the active-altruistic expression of his ego drives, as opposed to the active-egoistic expression. I will formally examine this in the next book when I re-introduce psychic bisexuality.

19 This sense of robbing or stealing from the phallic mother, or the reverse, will have different manifestations depending on the stage or level of authority that it concerns. The earlier the stage, the greater the magnitude.

20 To be a true parallel at the phallic stage, the primal scene in the object drives can merely be about one man "seducing" a woman into preferring him/loving him rather than another man. I have worked with several young men who have shown interest in a friend's girlfriend or vice versa. Sometimes while their friend is with the woman, or after they break up, the friend tries to date her. There are still very big feelings attached to feeling one's romantic partner loves another even if there is no cheating. Additionally, the strength of the humiliation and inferiority involved could place this primal scene in the ego drives at different levels as well. It is one thing to be humiliated at one's place of work, but the magnitude increases greatly if the humiliation is televised and everyone in society gets to view it.

21 I have to thank Dr. Michael Williams for tirelessly pointing this out to me.

22 When running outpatient substance abuse groups, I sometimes encounter an addict who has made it through residential treatment and can use treatment jargon very well. He can say some eloquent things, give good advice to others, but he either does not get personal or one can tell that he is using well-worn personal stories without giving something new about himself. He can be very helpful in the group but sometimes gets others to focus on him as the center of power more than the facilitator. He sometimes seems to set himself up as a would-be mentor to someone who is struggling and wants guidance. In individual therapy, I always begin with a history and when I do so, I often work with both by complimenting the patient or expressing surprise that he did not become more successful or recognized in his life, or by agreeing with him about the idiocy in the world. Once you give this "mirroring" to the patient, or "join his defense," as Hyman Spotnitz (1969) calls it, the patient can begin to get more personal and bring up his anxieties and inferiority feelings on his own. As opposed to trying to give one the impression that he does not have personal problems. Sometimes he will begin to bring you into his more personal thoughts of envy, reactivity, and discuss the "haters" in his life.

6

DISCUSSION 2

The impersonal and superpersonal imago and group psychology

In *The Economics of Libido* (2015) I introduce Freud's four levels of object relations development and try to sketch the different estimates of power in the imagos that comprise the mind. As explicated in Chapter 5, the difference between the generations in the phallic oedipal ego drives concerns how the individual recognizes parental-substitutes who possess more knowledge, skill, and Prestige, and those who pass these things on to neophytes in the community. From here, earlier imagos from the pre-phallic stages represent greater magnitudes of power. For example, there is a point at which Prestige switches over to the Superlative, so that one is driven to be the most powerful person, the smartest person, or to be at the top of social hierarchies. In Freud's four-stage model, this marks the transition from the phallic stage to the anal stage. In the next stage, the narcissistic stage, there are people who are viewed as more powerful than those at the anal stage in that they are felt to be semi-divine or superhuman. A king, for example, is seen as above regular humans, and as a figure to whom magical abilities are sometimes attributed, as well as some divine lineage. However, when one is not born a king, then one's skill, intelligence, and innovations can still grant the status of being immortal.[1] This means to become a great name who will always be remembered for his or her contributions to the arts, sciences, or historic events; this is in contrast to those who are at the top of hierarchies but can be forgotten in a few generations. Thus, being seen as knowledgeable or skilled in the community expands to being seen as "the best," to being "the best there ever was," and can still go to being God-like (as megalomania illustrates).

Along with the ways these imagos link to the depersonalized social body, with deepening levels of ambition as the example, there are also *impersonalized* and *superpersonalized* aspects to them.

For example, Freud (1930) expresses an important link between the impersonalization of the mother's body to an oceanic connection with the world. He writes of

> a feeling of an indissoluble bond, of being one with the external world as a whole . . . originally the ego includes everything, later it separates off an external world from itself. Our present ego-feeling is, therefore, only a shrunken residue of a much more inclusive—indeed, an all-embracing—feeling which corresponded to a more intimate bond between the ego and the world about it. If we may assume that there are many people in whose mental life this primary ego-feeling has persisted to a greater or less degree, it would exist in them side by side with the narrower and more sharply demarcated ego-feeling of maturity, like a kind of counterpart to it. In that case, the ideational contents appropriate to it would be precisely those of limitlessness and of a bond with the universe . . . the oceanic feeling, which might seek something like the restoration of limitless narcissism.
>
> *(pp. 65–72)*

The original "all-embracing" relation of the child to the mother becomes impersonalized as a relation to the world or external Space. Even before the earth was discovered to be a spherical planet in a solar system, there were early cultures that represented "the world" as being on a turtle's back or as being flat, for example. External Space can be an object upon which fantasies are externalized, disconnect with the external world can show up in pathology, and the contents of one's internal Space can rival external Space to preoccupy one's attention. As contrasted to later stages in which sexual and/or love feelings drive us to connections with others, at this stage the desire for a lover can be reduced to a masturbatory fantasy of one that is self-satisfied. In parallel, the desire for power can also be reduced to a fantasy of possessing it or as something vicariously experienced through movies.[2] I take this masturbatory aspect of internal Space to illustrate the basic set up of the first of Freud's four stages, *the auto-erotic stage.*

I would like to give a couple clinical examples to show interaction with Space as an imago:

> After her first few sessions, one client complains that she doesn't "feel real" and sometimes, conversely, has thoughts that the world isn't real. I ask her to focus on this feeling and begin BLS. She is able to get more in touch with the mindset and says that everything seems "hazy" and that her head feels "foggy." I ask her to focus on this again and resume BLS. Client expresses it differently, and says that she has the feeling of "flashing in and out of reality." I ask her to imagine someone or something that was flashing in and out of reality and put them in a "foggy and hazy place." She says she can picture a "boy in the woods" and that he is flashing in and out of world and that if he touches a tree that he would sometimes "phase through it." I ask her to make up a story and to tell me more about him. She says he is "sad, lost, and little." I ask her how he ended up in the woods all alone and who put this magical curse on him that was making him phase in and out of reality. She says that his mother was a drug addict and had "hid him in a crawlspace

in their house" and that he heard "traumatic events" and left the house and ran out to the woods. I note this, but because it seems autobiographical and could led her to events that she is not yet ready to face, I ask her to again picture the boy in the woods, phasing through trees and moving through the forest. I ask her to play this scene forward and to imagine what happens next. She says that a little unicorn comes along and that the boy sees it but "is not sure if he wants to follow it." I ask her to play it forward again and see what he does. She says that he follows alongside the unicorn, but that "he is not reaching out to see if it is real and "he doesn't know if it is real or in his own head." I ask her to play this forward again, and she says that "he walks side by side with it for years."

I ask her if his thoughts change and she says that he thinks about whether he will "accept or reject the purity [of the unicorn]" and that he thinks about "hugging it and never letting go." I ask her to describe his thoughts about it more and she says a few things that I put into object statements: "you're really pure, but you're going to disappear, you are too good to be true." I ask her to say these about someone from her past and see who shows up. She says that her "dad" comes to mind. She tells me that he died when she was 13 or 14 years old but that he "truly knew her" before he passed. She adds that her grandpa knew her too, but he had also died. She then says, "the only people who gave two fucks about me disappeared." I ask her to picture them and begin BLS again and ask her how they look to her. She cues me to stop and says that she feels sad and longs to be around them. I ask her to picture that she goes up to them and hugs them like the boy wanted to do with the unicorn, like she'll "never let them go." I begin BLS, and tears stream down her cheeks. I encourage her to let the sad boy come into her and let him have this moment as long as he needs it. She continues to cry. After she seems done, I ask her to focus on her body and to see what it feels like and I do another pass. She tells me that it feels like "a knot in her gut" has let go and that she feels relief. I ask her to focus on the relief and then to float back to a time when she remembered feeling like this. She tells me that it was gardening with her father when she was young. I ask her to picture as much detail in the memory that she can and then to let it come into her as much as she can. After BLS, I ask her how much she feels "in reality," or if she feels that things are hazy or foggy still and she says that they aren't, and she feels present.

Another client gives me a flying dream. He is an addict and when he mentions flying "high" I think of relating it to his addiction. However, when he begins talking about "not being limited by gravity" and "defying gravity," I begin to think about it on another track. I ask him to anthropomorphize gravity or, to be more precise, I ask him to pretend that gravity was controlled by a person, and what that person might think about him flying and "defying gravity." He says that this person might feel "bedazzled, curious, angry, embarrassed" (if he tries to fathom his reaction). I ask client to explain the

> reactions and he says, the man would probably think: "how is he doing this?" "I've never got to do this (get away with this as a kid)," and "He can't get away with this." We discuss potential envy feelings as well as the awe in the bedazzled adjective. I ask him to say these as ego and object statements and see who he has felt this relation with. He relates these feelings to "cops and judges," but then also mentions that his mother comes up and talks about how she didn't like him riding motorcycles and dirt bikes when he was young.

Whether it is one being in the world or feeling unreal, or entering into a rivalry with the laws of physics that govern the world, Space can be isolated as an imago. Once this is done, relations can be made to return the conflicts or absences found there to their interpsychic roots with parents or parental-substitutes. Although daydreamers and "space cases" are examples of pathology at this stage, fantasy, as Freud (1917c, p. 375) discusses it, is very important for both art and intellectualism. Instead of a connection to one's body and/or the bodies of others in external Space, one's internal world, or internal Space, is valorized. Whether it is rehashing one's memories, or forming them into daydreams, stories, or cataloguing them, the "mind's eye" can receive a great economical significance (i.e. receive more attention or energy than other things in one's life). Along with artists and intellectuals who valorize internal Space, there are scientists and others who valorize external Space and solitary pursuits of empiricism in the environment or in the lab. Fairbairn (1952) sees both aspects as schizoid,

> that intellectual pursuits as such, whether literary, artistic, scientific, or otherwise, appear to exercise a special attraction for individuals possessing schizoid characteristics to one degree or another. Where scientific pursuits are concerned, the attraction would appear to depend upon the schizoid individual's attitude of detachment no less than upon his overvaluation of the thought-processes; for these are both characteristics which readily lend themselves to capitalization within the field of science. The obsessional appeal of science, based as this is upon the presence of a compulsive need for orderly arrangement and meticulous accuracy, has, of course, long been recognized; but the schizoid appeal is no less definite and demands at least equal recognition. Finally the statement may be hazarded that a number of outstanding historical figures lend themselves to the interpretation that they were either schizoid personalities or schizoid characters; and indeed it would appear as if it were often such who leave a mark upon the page of history.
>
> *(p. 6)*

The "attitude of detachment" in schizoid phenomena also applies to those preoccupied with the non-human environment, animals, physics, etc., and who spend more time thinking about these things, than about human relations. A scientist in a lab, a ranger who makes solitary rounds in a state park, or someone coding on a computer all day are examples of people who illustrate this detachment. However, as with the artist, these work object-choices can also be influenced by one's parents, other parental-substitutes, and inputs from later stages of development; one cannot assume deutero adaptations or fixations without seeing other evidence. Additionally, there is also an important question of defusion, defenses, and schizoid pathology, which can make such professions salient because one feels uncomfortable being around other human bodies. As mentioned in Chapter 2, the sense of how much intellectual activities are part of one's being is the issue for the deutero phase.

Although ordering the contents of Space is important for intellectual creativity and innovation, genius requires a great memory. He or she must synthesize new ideas from all the available data or borrow an analogy from some other facet of life.[3] This ability to synthesize well is predicated on an excellent memory, both as remembering the past and being able to learn new things by having a good attention span. Memory and attention span can hugely vary between people and in classical psychoanalysis Klein (1932) refers to it as the epistemophilic drive and connects it with the first Oedipus complex and the "maximal sadism" of the infant (p. 99 fn, 242). Along with inhibitions in learning, Klein (1931) also describes pathology at this stage that shows

> the effect of this inhibition [to] the whole attitude to the external world and impair[ed] orientation in its widest and most metaphorical sense . . . this inhibition is due to fear of the mother's body, in consequence of sadistic attacks upon it, and has also demonstrated that the early sadistic phantasies about the mother's body and a capacity to work these over successfully form the bridge to object-relationships and adaptation to reality, thus fundamentally influencing the subject's later relation to the external world.
>
> *(p. 212 fn)*

A person's natural sense of direction in Space can be lost in psychopathology. The relation to external Space can take on the ambivalence that one feels towards a parent (or substitute). As mentioned in earlier chapters, Freud (1914a, 1919b, 1921) also gives us examples of the projection of cognitive functions into external Space so that an individual can be overly related to the world, and feel that it is looking back at him. I anticipate that psychopathology like hoarding and ADHD will be found to involve a relation to the impersonal imago of Space too. Additionally, in Chapter 2, I gave a clinical example of the double in which my patient described his "world on fire," which illustrates another relation to this imago. Despite the power of this fantasy, which issued from PI with the castrated phallic mother imago, my patient had no complaints of relating to external Space. Instead, this PI was linked to self-sabotage in which any attempts to gain a good name, a family, and have the good things that others possess, were foiled by his own impulsive misdeeds. He was dependent on living with family, had nothing of his own, and kept finding himself at this place of being a "zero."

In "Attacks on Linking" (1959), Bion carries on the Kleinian paradigm and brings in the dimension of the impersonalized relation to internal Space in the form of affect block. He holds that

> the refusal of the mother to serve as a repository for the infant's feelings, or by the hatred and envy of the patient who cannot allow the mother to exercise this function, leads to a destruction of the link between infant and breast and consequently to a severe disorder of the impulse to be curious on which all learning depends. The way is therefore prepared for a severe arrest of development. Furthermore, thanks to a denial of the main method open to the infant for dealing with his too powerful emotions, the conduct of emotional life, in any case a severe problem, becomes intolerable. Feelings of hatred are thereupon directed against all emotions including hate itself, and against external reality which stimulates them. It is a short step from hatred of the emotions to hatred of life itself.
>
> *(p. 314)*

Bion links the perception of external Space, which includes a drive to record information (curiosity), with the relation to one's own body and the mother's, and how both can be defended against. The standard schizoid personality disorder will see the sacrifice of the object drive relation of his body to another's, so that there is an affect block and no registered desire for a relationship.[4] The stereotype here is someone like Mr. Spock on *Star Trek* in which the individual often speaks about what is logical, is flat in affect, and gives off a sense of cold indifference. However, it is also possible that the ego drives and attention span are defended against and you can have an impulsive person who is exclusively focused on object drives, has no attention span, and bears little resemblance to an intellectual schizoid. Additionally, there are people in PI at this stage who feel as though they must appear as god-like, and can never admit to, or apologize for their mistakes. Their grandiosity, in many cases, is not overt and is only perceived indirectly, by the way their internal Space makes them so sensitive to any criticisms. In contrast, I have also worked with passive-altruists who feel like they must be mind readers and anticipate the desires of their parent (or substitute) in an omnipotent way, and have a symbiotic relation to the internal Space of their object.

Along with Space as an imago, with both external and internal aspects, the world often appears as the creation of a god and a superpersonal relation to Him is possible. God features prominently in the narratives of many patients with primitive superego issues. One such patient discussed with me how the Devil's mistake was that he tried to take God's power and never simply asked God to give him a planet to control. My patient expressed the desire to have a world to take care of and for the population to love him. With some analysis, he was able to articulate that he would give the people mana from heaven, that they would feel gratitude towards him, and that they would probably worship him. However, this led to explicit competition with God (i.e. God reserves the sole right to be worshipped). His fantasy shifted to the idea that God would not just want to watch creation, and would want to live and experience His own creation by becoming human. My patient shared "secret knowledge," that he was "God in the flesh who wants to live life," and sometimes tried to focus his will to access his Godly power (ex. "I think what I want and

POOF it is there"). In later sessions, he talked about "begging" God to bless his relationship with a woman and protect his love with her. He expressed his frustration with Him as "I care about you, I love you, why don't you treat me better?" I asked him to put this into ego and object statements and he said his mother came to mind and got into how "she should have done a lot more things" for him and feelings of disappointment with her.

For many patients who have lived through major traumas, God is the repository of their ambivalence with parents (or substitutes). He can be as disappointing as people, and they can consciously be angry with Him for having let terrible things happen to them. This is important to work through before any higher-level issues, in my experience. For solely verbal psychotherapy, God and supernatural figures are often the simplest way to access the earliest levels of development. Along with such figures, in Chapter 2 I showed that relations to inanimate things, animals, sleep, etc. can also express the ego injuries of interpsychic conflicts, and are a port of entry for early levels of development. Thus, it is also important to recognize that every stage has different displacement objects that can be the basis of symptoms and comprise a *subpersonalized* imago relation. Lacan (1998) has a contribution to make here in the relation of his concept of object *a* to feces, for example, instead of to the bodily zone of the anus. The bodily zones themselves are very important and related to the production of symbols, as shown in Chapter 2, but the subpersonal objects related to the zones can also be areas of intense focus for the unconscious. More discussions on the subpersonal and displaceables (i.e. animals, inanimate objects, etc.) will take place in the next book.

In *The Economics of Libido* (2015), I link Time with the stage following the auto-erotic, *the narcissistic stage.*

Just as there are hallucinations that show the confusion between internal and external Space, Freud (1909b, 1913) found that some people experienced bad conscience from the negative wishes that they had towards others. He calls this phenomenon "the omnipotence of wishes" and it should be understood as being mediated by Time. Freud (1913) links the omnipotence of wishes to animistic religions of the past, but this egocentrism is still around today in books like *The Secret* (Byrne, 2008), or practices like Reiki healing, among others. These practices are predicated on a belief that one's wishes are taken to cause success, destruction, or healing. In contrast to regarding one's will or love as causing effects without any visible indicators, active hallucinatory illusions such as flying or a wizard conjuring something into existence out of nothing, have a greater magnitude and fit better in the auto-erotic stage.

Chapter 2 addresses how Rank and Freud invoke the importance of immortality in relation to a subjective sense of death. Although immortality is often linked to the religious afterlife and magic, which register at the auto-erotic stage, I will provide some clinical examples that illustrate the importance of Time at a lesser magnitude than this. The omnipotence of wishes references that a person either cares enough about external Time to actually study the efficacy of his wishes, or he privileges his own internal sense of Time. Although we share social conventions for telling time in regards to the 12-hour clocks, it must not be forgotten that we also possess a subjective sense of Time. Meissner (2008) collects relevant writing from many philosophical, psychological, and neurological sources to express views that Time can fly by, drag on, or stand still for different people at different moments. Beyond different forms of measuring time, the concept of external Time requires some shared sense of being "in sync" with humanity and some basic form of shared social organization.

In a very suggestive article, Loewald (1962) theorizes that the relation of the superego agency to the ego agency as one that is related temporally. He writes:

> Insofar as the superego is the agency of inner standards, demands, ideals, hopes and concerns in regard to the ego, the agency of inner rewards and punishments in respect to which the ego experiences contentment or guilt, the superego functions from the viewpoint of a future ego, from the standpoint of the ego's future which is to be reached, is being reached, is being failed or abandoned by the ego.
>
> *(p. 265)*

In working with chemical dependence, one can see a complete disregard for the future of the ego that Loewald mentions. Many addicts have not seen a dentist or doctor for years and have secret fears that they have a disease or have done irreparable harm to themselves. Their present is often filled with every kind of distraction and form of procrastination so that they do not perceive their future nor feel the demands of their ego ideal. Loewald differentiates phases of the superego and posits "magical communion with an ideal authority" in early development and also mentions the child satisfying itself with hallucinatory wish fulfillment (ibid., p. 266). However, he does not mention any progression to the omnipotence of wishes, nor does he provide any examples of pathology that showcase how an early phase issue with the imago may affect the general relation to Time. Regardless, an important seed was planted with observing a temporal relation in the superego.

Eigen (1983), in a short essay on time in dreams, discusses Time in ways that apply to both dreams and real life. "[D]reams handle time in as many ways as there are defensive styles," he writes, which "reflect the dreamer's changing time experience in novel and clarifying ways" (ibid., p. 219). In his ideas of "lived time" and "ways of relating to time," Eigen importantly hints at underlying psychodyamics. In another essay, "The Recoil on Having Another Person" (1993), he gives the interesting case of man gripped by self-sabotage in business and who ran through a large number of friendships. Eigen is able to connect success in these realms as "closing possibilities, ending distance, while in failing, [his patient] could seem to be always starting anew" (ibid., p. 23). Friends that represented a future and therefore "temporal integration" were avoided and Eigen emphasized the "temporal meaning" of relationships (ibid., p. 24). The basic insight of temporal meaning organizing relationships and being caught up in psychodynamics is here.

Kavaler-Adler (2013) brings in both psychopathology and the idea of immortality in her discussion of Time as an object. She follows in the Freudian and Rankian tradition of noting the mediation of immortality and mortality through Time, and ties her insight to an enlarged conception of Winnicott's transitional space and transitional object. However, her views of immortality are more informed by Deprak Chopa, whom she cites, than by Freudian metapsychology or primary narcissism, which are not mentioned. The "dialectic between mortality and immortality," she writes, is related to "time . . . as holding and filled with infinite possibilities rather than as linear and persecutory" (p. 28). Examples of persecutory experiences of Time are problems with time management (i.e. fear of deadlines) and being unable to be in the moment while dancing. She also mentions having to face becoming old or patients "killing time" instead of being emotionally open in session because of a lack of trust. Kavaler-Adler's formulations are often impressionistic and do not reference any systematic sense of the imago in question. Still, she echoes Eigen's insight that Time relates to psychodynamics and more explicitly points to the internal object or imago as the central concern.

In classical literature, Reich (1990) and other analysts have written about compulsive characters who are compared to "living machines" and bring up coordinates of a human vs. non-human distinction. There are famous stories of the philosopher Kant, for example, going for walks at the same time every day, despite the weather, and being extremely regular in all things. Others could set their watch or clock by his daily passing and the obviously eccentric nature of this shows how he is machine-like in comparison to "regular humans." A reference to shared, external Time and being in synch with humanity is the foundational reference to the imago of Time. In contrast, some of the resistances that patients show in the session (ex. being emotionally closed off), or outside of the session (ex. problems getting in to work on time) can reference many other issues that have nothing to do with the global relation to the Time imago. For example, in Chapter 5 we saw Mcdougall's example of procrastination as the conversion of anxiety with a patient who otherwise showed good structure in his life (i.e. had a job, kept appointments, etc.). In the next book, I will formally discuss self-sabotage and how issues with deadlines relate to an economics of punishment or apathy.

I would like to give a couple clinical examples that show this relation to the imago of Time:

> Client brings up self-criticism and problems with procrastination due to feelings that he should live with every moment of his day scheduled. He reports feeling like he should get up early in the morning and be totally prepared for work; he should not eat out and shop so much and save money; he should go fishing on weekends because he should do something he likes, etc. However, client reports that he often pushes the snooze button and tells himself "five more minutes" (which usually turns into an hour). Client also reports buying new things despite his aspirations for money management,

and talks about how he talks himself into staying in town or to do projects at home rather than fish or engage in hobbies. But, rather than doing all the things on his list and scheduled timeline, he says he often ends up watching YouTube videos and doing nothing. I formally introduce the conflict in him as involving a procrastinating part of himself and a tyrannical time-manager who is obsessed with the ideal use of Time. I ask him to talk about the relation between these two parts and he says that former is "clever" and sees the latter part as "weak and irritating." I ask him to put these into ego and object statements (i.e. "you are weak, you are irritating, I am clever") and he tells me that his father comes to mind. Client goes on to explain that his father was weak because he "lacked conviction" and was irritating because he said he cared about him and his brother and would be around more, but never was. Client's anger is palpable as he talks about his father and he begins to discharge it in swearing about his father.

Another client missed his previous session and had missed another one before. Instead of just treating this as transference, I tried to determine if this was a way of Being for him. Usually it's not difficult to tell if the patient is regressed, and living day to day— hour to hour is often more precise in some cases—because the client doesn't have a job and is usually manic or depressed. This client has a job, is in a long-term relationship, and is more functional. However, he does admit to part of him feeling like he lives day to day and is just "going through the motions" in his life. He reports that he sometimes misses appointments with other professionals, simply forgets plans he had made, and doesn't have any apparatus in place for scheduling things out of his normal daily routine. I begin to build a metaphor with him. I tell client that he has an interesting relationship to Time and that outside of the daily routine, it was like he expected Time to take care of him, and remind him of any special occasions that he might forget. I compare it to how I let my mother wake me up for school without setting an alarm for myself as a teen. He accepts the metaphor, and I ask him to tell me his thoughts about how Time sometimes fails him and "doesn't remind him of his appointments." This way of looking at things resonates with him, and he says that it's like Time "dropped the ball," "was forgetful herself," and that he feels "disappointed" when she "fails" him. I ask client to say these as ego and object statements: "you dropped the ball, you are forgetful, you disappointed me, you failed me." Client tells me his mother comes to mind. He says that his grandmother was more of a mom than his mother was: his mother "hadn't been a mother" and "didn't do her job." Client gets into particular moments of her using and selling drugs and being caught up in the lifestyle. We analyze them and he gets in touch with strong disappointment with her. However, instead of becoming anger it becomes idealization and client says, "she's better than how she was acting." I begin BLS and ask him to picture her at the time when she had been acting irresponsibly and to tell her everything that he told me and then to see how she looks. After BLS,

> he signals me to stop and says that her inner representation "took" what he had to say. He reports new feelings of being "more proud of her now" and says that "she's back to what she should be." He even expresses, spontaneously, that if he shared these thoughts with her that "she'd probably cry." I investigate possible resistance for client to act on this impulse but he doesn't seem to feel any and declares that he is going to say something to her when he gets up to leave at the end of the session.

Time is taken as an imago in these examples and my patients' relations to others become globally affected. In the first example, my patient had a compulsive symptom of ideal time management, which he obsessed about, and rebelled against, in his solitary existence. With the latter patient, there was a passive dependence in his impersonal relation to Time that repeated an ego injury from a parent and kept him open to the feeling of further neglect.[5] These examples show that a person can leave the realm of a structured or higher-functioning lifestyle and enter a realm in which they are out of sync with other humans and ambivalent about their connections to others and society in general.

The superpersonal at this stage is best related to the idea of obsession or fascination with the Timeless. As God creates the world or external Space and can become a major focus of some patients, external Time must similarly be ordered by a principle. As mentioned, there are those whose ambition is to be "the best there has ever been" and to be Timeless or immortal. This goes along with obsession in their field of work. For such people, this fascination takes precedence above any human relation. Some of the addicts I work with do not just have an auto-erotic relation to their drug, in which they want to control their experience of consciousness or defend against unwanted feelings or ideas. Some of them also discuss drugs as a way of life: one in which they have a reason to relate to others and without which they feel awkward, like weird outsiders, failures, or losers. For other patients, the fixation on the superpersonal Timeless is a magical historical era that is decisively not our current era. Some patients have shared thoughts on how things were perfect in the 1960s, how they should have been born in medieval times, or how some other time was the best things ever were. The "magical" or semi-supernatural flavor that the Timeless has, can shift between individual examples, as can the sense of glory or harmony of the people there. For example, with one young patient, there was a valorization of ancient Rome and a reported disconnect with other "humans" of his time. A strong sense of death came up in the fantasy he constructed:

> Client had dropped out of college and then gets into a history of quitting things. He tells me about how he stopped playing hockey when he was in middle school to the chagrin of his parents. He uses the expression "two sides clashing" to talk about the opposition from his parents on such decisions, and I ask him to associate to this phrase. He says it reminds him of two sides in a war. I ask him for the first war that came to his mind and he says a war in ancient Rome. I ask him to picture a war from this period and describe what

> his imagination lays out before him. He does so and then begins focusing on "the bunch of people in the back waiting for war." Client explains how the war happens in the front lines, and that for many soldiers it is a matter of "just waiting." I ask client what kind of mood they seem to be in while they are just waiting? He says that they are "sighing," and thinking, "What are we doing here?" I ask him to imagine what they are thinking as they move closer to the front, and he says that they are thinking that they are "closer to death" and "feel anxious." I ask what happens when they finally make it to the front, and he laughs uncomfortably and says that he imagines that they kill the other side. However, he quickly adds that he doesn't like it, although he identifies with them, and is "on their side." I ask him what happens after they are victorious and he says that they are "tired, down-faced, and had enough of this." I ask him to imagine what they look like and he says they have slumping shoulders because they "just killed a bunch of people and weren't feeling good about it." I ask him to put the first part of this into ego statements ("I am tired, down-faced, and have had enough of this") and to see if they feel true for a part of him. He says that they do and then adds that he feels "detachment from the world" and "doesn't enjoy what most people do." He quickly adds that the last statement "sounds bad," but I encourage him to talk more. He complains about "reality stars" and their "drama" and how these ancient soldiers had a much more "meaningful existence." He says that they built the longest roads in history in the Roman Empire and soldiers worked alongside slaves but "didn't care about social status." He tells me that they were "more goal-oriented" and discusses more of their project. I ask about how the upper-class people treated the slaves and he says that they had "more of an ego," and were "snobby and impatient." I ask him to turn these adjectives into object statements and he associates to his parents first, and then brings up being a "nerd" in middle school and associates to his experience on sports teams and a particularly mean girl.

My patient's Timeless object of fascination goes along with a withdrawal of ego interest from others, but not as severe as in psychosis, of course. Interestingly, I have also seen the opposite phenomenon with some of the addicts I work with. Sometimes, their drug use allows them to valorize their connection with fellow users to create the sense that they are having "the best night ever," or that their friendships or romances are the ideal. Gamblers or addicts of various types can make their lives revolve around their obsession and can potentially lose everything else (money, family, friendships, love, etc.). Similarly, workaholics can burn through several marriages and families even though they keep their success and wealth. Functionally, these types are pursuing something that is greater than human relationships, with the irony that they sometimes believe that the object of fascination will bring them the relationships they want, while it is what pushes others away. Again, people at this level show more relatedness to others than someone in psychosis, but their relatedness is more accurately designated by the idea of pseudo-relations. I say pseudo-relations because many addicts will have complaints that their "friends" never wrote or visited them in jail, their "friends" often lied, stole from them, or used them, and things were far from ideal. When these patients became incarcerated, the party went on without them, and when they were no longer there to live in the moment, they were easily forgotten. The Timeless object that takes one out of human relationships can put one on a path of not just becoming eccentric but non-human and monstrous. I hope this does not come across as moralizing on my part, because my patients taught me to use words like monstrous. This moral concern will come into greater relief when I discuss group psychology below.

At the anal stage, loving feelings in the object drives and desire for role-based identity in the ego drives enter psychosexual development for the active-egoist. "Defaecation" Freud (1917e) writes, "affords the first occasion on which the child must decide between a narcissistic [ego drive] and an object-loving attitude" (p. 130). Although full affectionate love enters the active pole in the phallic stage, the anal stage can display powerful, passionate love. In the ego drives, one is firmly chasing success and the imperative to be the best in the power hierarchies of external Civilization. This is contrasted with internal Civilization, in which members of organized crime groups, for example, rival the laws of Civilization with their own laws. In organized crime, members may be permitted to murder, steal, and traffic drugs so long as such acts do not transgress the laws of their new "family." Different subcultures may not emphasize illegality as much in variations of psychic bisexuality; "hipsters," "neo-hippies," and other groups emphasize certain aesthetics and consumption patterns that make them visibly inhabit a role or lifestyle choice. So long as members of such groups are not radical and accept the legitimacy of the ruling structure of society, then the imago of Civilization is the focus for people who are ambivalent about regular "civilian," "tax-paying," or "consumer" lifestyles.

This level of Being often shows up in many of the criminal patients with whom I work. There is often a sense of a wealthier, more educated class from which they are excluded. For example:

> One client gets into sensations related to feeling like he's "falling apart." We work with sensations in his heart, throat, and tongue and introject pencils and other symbols to get past his affect blocks. Interestingly, after the pencil is fully embedded, it clears out the sensations of tightness in his tongue and throat and client feels the energy from this zone go to his stomach. We turn to his chest. I ask him to project out the sensation there and he tells me that he pictures "wrapped gauze" that is "about the width of two fingers" and he also compares it to being "mummy wrapped." When there is a sense of some tension in a projected image or there is a sense of something being covered or hidden, I always ask the patient to take the image to the next stage and tell me what happens or what is revealed. In this case, client tells me that he pictures two pens inside the mummy wrap. I ask him to describe them and he says that they are "expensive" and "fatter" and have "gold trim." I ask him

> who he pictures that they might belong to. Client says "office types" and the first person who comes to mind is his son's mother. He tells me about her office job. I ask him to talk more about office types and how he relates to this class of people. He quickly says that he feels "accepted by every class" but then adds that "it didn't use to be like that." I ask him to associate to when he wasn't accepted by them and he tells me that before he went to prison the was a "punk" and was "disrespectful to authority." He then brings up his ex-girlfriend's father and an officer in the prison. I ask him to picture these two men and see who figures more prominently to him and begin BLS. He tells me that the officer does. He explains that this officer put him in the hole "for dumb shit" and was a "dick" and had "power and control issues." I ask him to focus on this officer and to see what time with him comes to mind the most and resume BLS. He tells me that he was in the hole one time and was asking for something and "he was not giving it to [him] at all." I ask him to focus on this, resume BLS, and he tells me that he feels anger coming up. I tell him to stay with it, see how it wants to be expressed in his body. After he ascertains this, I then tell him to picture the officer in the hole with him and begin with his words and then see if his body wants him to do more. I begin BLS, and when he signals that he's done, he tells me that he kicked him in the chest, called him a "nigger," and that officer was "on the ground, bloody." I ask him to focus on him on the ground, all bloody, and see if his body has a reaction to this. After BLS, he reports that more calm came in to his body.[6]

The sense of being judged by others for both one's criminal past and for re-entering Civilization in a low-paying job is often a major impediment for active-egoists. They cannot tolerate that others are looking at them like they are a "piece of shit" and often try to convince me that it is better for them to go back to prison and "kill their number" than it is to put up with the rules of, and judgments from probation officers, the halfway house, or the average citizen.[7] Sometimes they do not simply view themselves as being lower class or beneath tax-paying citizens ("normies"), but instead they believe that they are part of a subculture that should be the dominant culture, or that represents what is best in Civilization. They often think about themselves as the "true Americans," for example, who have common sense, the proper work ethic, and the right sense for how things should be.

The anal stage is the first stage of secondary narcissism. The stages of primary narcissism concern ways of life that are linked to worldviews that surround immortality (an afterlife/the supernatural) or some view of a perfect, Timeless place. In contrast, the anal stage concerns lifestyles that accept the basic authority in society but may also maintain a belief that the values associated with their roles, or lifestyles should be the ones that govern Civilization. I do not want to give the sense that this belief only exists within antisocial or anti-authoritarian subcultures. There are many people who see their profession (i.e. lawyer, banker, psychologist) as also suggesting a role that they should play in society, and exemplifying certain values that should have more governing force in Civilization.

The superpersonal dimension often comes up with patients as the System and relates to the elite who are in control of it. External Civilization is created or governed by the elite who make the rules for different systems within society. For example, those who are caught up in the legal system can have the sense that it is unfair to them, skewed in the favour of certain people, is oppressive, or designed to make them fail. One criminal patient railed against "the system," and I elicited adjectives about it: "flawed, changing, broken, and corrupt." He was able to say them as both ego and object statements and recognized a part of him that was like this, as well as seeing these qualities in his absent, addicted father. Having to join his father in "cheap, crackhead motels" and witnessing his lies about using needles for diabetes when he was clearly high and paranoid created an ego injury. This became connected to the self-sabotage of his goals so that he would repeat his father's life: "stuck in a dead end job, and not happy," and with the sense that he "should have tried harder."[8] External Civilization can be broken down into many systems at the anal level, and whether one has concerns with systemic racism on the left, a system that is impinging on personal freedoms on the right, or general principles about how businesses, schools, etc. should function, there is the possibility that ego injuries and fantasies can be externalized onto these systems.

Lastly, I have already mentioned the phallic community in relation to the depersonalized imago and its relevance regarding reputation. However, the phallic Family better captures what is at stake in the impersonalized imago at this level. The external Family concerns things such as birth to biological parents and one's literal procreators, but in a wider sense it also includes "the village" it takes to raise a child. External Family is issued by "accidental" or pre-determined factors regarding where and to whom one was born. An internal Family arises from people having the sense that they have chosen friends, colleagues, or intimates to be around them like a family (or, at least have not chosen to leave them). The superpersonal aspect here is Fate or that which has ordered those things that have come into one's life by chance. Freud (1930) writes:

> In the original infantile stage of conscience, which, as we see, is not given up after the introjection into the super-ego, but persists alongside of it and behind it[,] Fate is regarded as a substitute for the parental agency. If a man is unfortunate it means that he is no longer loved by this highest power; and, threatened by such a loss of love, he once more bows to the parental representative in his super-ego—a representative whom, in his days of good fortune, he was ready to neglect.
>
> *(pp. 126–127)*

This sense of Fate can surely register at other levels, and show up, for example, in how some people are angry at God for what happened to them. However, I tie it to the phallic stage specifically because of the way that some patients are fixated on how their Family is seen in the community and how this reflects on them. They talk about others who come from good families and convey a sense of how they are unfairly judged for their origins. Conversely, in some triangles, the "other man" with whom one competes for recognition, or a romantic partner, can be envied or denigrated for the backing he gets from Family. For example, one male patient repeatedly found himself in relationships in which his love object would leave him for another man. As a means to work through this pattern, I asked him to generally describe the common traits that these men have had. My patient described this other man as "like [him] but [he] has stuff out of my reach," "he has his shit together," and "he lived the life that I had my goals set to live." This patient was able to associate to others from his past who were not involved in the love triangles. One was a cousin who he complained "had more opportunities than [him]" and my patient talked about how he had a car that he had been fixing up, but then his uncle had bought his cousin the same car outright. His focus was on how his cousin "had a backing that [he] didn't have."

One of the many surprises that I have had in the clinic is to see the great ego injury that some patients experienced when they found out that they were adopted. Although their adopted parents treated them well and were functionally their parents in every way, to find that Fate played some cruel joke or put them where they did not belong was a major shock for them. Like my other clinical examples, this does not come from some guess, or interpretation, but from patients associating to ego and object statements, bodily gestures, or feeling states. To be clear, this does not show up as an ego injury with every patient who was adopted or raised by someone else, just as one sibling could have PTSD from sexual abuse even though the other sibling who got the same treatment does not have it.

I

The previous chapter examined the deutero phase in the phallic stage. However, as mentioned, the phallic mother and combined-parent imagos, exist at other stages, as do primal scenes.[9] The phallic mother offers the active-egoist a phallic image to approximate and an ability to inspire others as someone who is "cool" or charismatic. He or she is someone who others would want for a boss or to *lead* them, which is not based upon them being the most skilled or competent. He or she possesses attractive confidence from being loved by, or being like the phallic mother. Other stages would similarly give the individual power from the paternal imago, but, as mentioned in Chapter 5, Kohut's etiology of narcissistic issues from lack of parental mirroring suggests another potential cause of the deutero phase (Kohut, 1971). It is possible that the phase and the phallic mother may be formed from a rejecting or indifferent phallic mother imago at other stages. Additionally, it is possible that the low ego ideal might not register as attractive confidence in all of these stages, even though the deutero individual may still "give an impression of greater force and of more freedom of libido" (Freud, 1921, p. 130). Many patients who seem to have anal deutero character, for example, come off as more intimidating or brooding and less social than their phallic counterparts.

At the anal deutero phase, the individual would inspire others as someone to *command* or govern them. Instead of just impressing them as "cool," there would be the impression of more power in the individual. As mentioned in Chapter 5, Lowen (1994) connects the psychopathic character to the anal stage and holds that certain physical traits, such as a puffed-up chest, would go along with the deutero phase here.[10] Anyway, wanting to be "the boss" or in charge, seems more significant in my experience of the anal deutero phase. In contrast, the phallic deutero character does not attack the leader for control, in my experience, so much as attract attention away from him or her. In pathology, the phallic deutero character ends up seeming "slick," "too polished," and the attractive confidence gives way to vanity. In contrast, the anal deutero types are the ones who are either much more openly critical and dismissive or brooding and private.

The deutero narcissistic phase creates a type that inspires others as semi-divine, regal, noble-blooded, and gives the impression that he or she should *rule*. Again, this impression does not come from competency and experience, but through a low ego ideal, which can sometimes be expressed as "lordly affectation" in its pathological or sloppy expression (Reich, 1990, pp. 195–198). Clinically, I have very mixed counter-transference with narcissistic deutero types, and nothing conclusive to write. It is likely that there are different stages that are more libidinal, and stages that are more aggressive in their deutero phase manifestations, but I need more data at this point. In lieu of it, I will contain this discussion within the framework of observations regarding how the deutero type expresses a larger magnitude of power at earlier levels and that patients of this type, and those around them, often use aristocratic language to express their ability to inspire.

At the auto-erotic stage, the last expression of leadership is to fully *possess* the other. This follows from Freud's discussion of the hypnotist in the ego ideal, and also invokes the magnitude of "the devils" that show up in clinical work (Freud, 1921; Fairbairn, 1952). The low ego ideal gives the impression that one can rival Space or "the world," and the deutero type here gives the impression that his internal world houses as much as the external world. This person may appear as a "brain" with dictionary-like knowledge, or as though he could live alone on a mountaintop without being lonely or going crazy. As with comparing someone to a king or queen, some borderline patients often compare their romantic partners to God or accuse them of behaving like they are a god. Similarly, some artists and intellectuals have disclosed how their pursuits take them into "the essence of things," or are comparable to "decoding reality," thus implying a rivalry with God or a sense of taking His secrets.

We have already seen how these levels of authority show different estimates of power in the human and non-human environment, and provide a reference to different levels of ambition. However, each level also has its own form of group psychology as Freud (1921) investigates. These are best referenced in regards to different forms of aggression. In *The Economics of Libido* (2015), I follow Freud (1915a) in discussing the progression of sadism from destructive impulses concerning the body alone, to the sadism that is expressed in verbal attacks against a person's image or reputation (p. 128). Again, having one's reputation attacked in the community is the social anxiety of the phallic stage. This concerns one's competency, misdeeds, or character and depending on the seriousness or the magnitude of the charges, such an attack may register at earlier levels of development. In contrast, anal sadism is a more egocentric construction than the image-ego. It expresses more empathy for what is going on in the mind of others, and therefore arises later in development for the active-egoist, but the sadism is of a greater magnitude and therefore is earlier than the phallic stage. In my clinical experience, I often see anal sadism expressed with the idea that death for an ex-romantic partner or enemy is "too easy." These patients spin out involved revenge fantasies of wanting to watch those that wronged them "lose everything good in their lives" and "suffer a long, miserable life alone." However, like attacks on reputation entering into deeper levels, so can sadism enter deeper levels so that attacks on the body in torture, for example, can be enjoyed.

In the shift from secondary narcissism to primary narcissism the objectivity of knowing the consequences of the acts of aggression is not available to the child. In Chapter 2, the aim to cause someone's death (i.e. murder) was contrasted with the subjective death involved in primary narcissism. The former is part of the anal stage, along with anal sadism, while the latter is part of the narcissistic stage. Subjective death, as with annihilation aggression in the auto-erotic stage, references the subjective experience of losing psychic and somatic integrity, and reversing this experience to give the same to someone else. As mentioned, these can be paired with the intentional states of the higher stages of development. Additionally, along with a reference to specific bodily zones (ex. cannibalism and orality) the aggressive impulses can also reference technological advances like using bombs and explosives that would objectively cause the specific type of anxiety.

These different types of aggression provide a trans-historical starting point for the social anxiety surrounding the ethical life of humans, which also has inputs for specific historical laws and mores. Complicated moral ideas, or a fully reasoned ethical system, are not required to prove the wrongness of murder, for example. Rather, the subjective feelings of the id impulse to kill the anal parental imago is prohibited because it is associated with the superior power of the parents. However, a Janus-faced aspect is clearly present here. While some earlier political economies may have allowed revenge killing, for example, it is something that is outlawed in more developed ones. Thus, along with whatever impulses are prohibited in relation to parental-substitutes at the anal stage, there is also structural system of discourse that adds content to the laws of Civilization and ethical life. It is an object of sociological study to show how such laws have become linked to the social anxiety of imagos, and sociologists like Norbert Elias (1994), have done very interesting work in this field.

While the social anxiety of the phallic stage concerns folkways that comprise norms of politeness and decency, we can identify the anal imago with the police and the threat of prison, or being seen as a criminal in our current political economy. For anyone who works with criminals, the police are major transference figures, but even in therapy groups I sometimes become set up as someone who must defend the logic of laws and what members see as an unfair system. Other analysts have also noted a connection between anality and certain criminal acts, or with the legal system itself. For example, Klein (1975, pp. 142, 228) adds robbery as a destructive act associated with anality, and Erik Erikson (1963, p. 254) formally links the anal stage to "the principle of law and order."

There are still levels of social anxiety that have greater magnitude in entering primary narcissism. Certain crimes are not merely criminal and can give one the reputation of being "monstrous." A good prototype for this greater level of shame are oral-cannibalistic impulses, which have an instinctual basis. While criminal activities like robbery or murder are criminal, one can still understand them as human failings. Cannibalism, however, presents the idea of something not just criminal, but almost incomprehensible. In fairy tales, monsters and witches are often attributed with a desire to eat humans and their supernatural nature also points to the deeper magnitude of this level. However, this level also has inputs for the discourse from a particular political economy. For example, certain religious symbols can become sacred in a culture and their desecration can be seen as monstrous. Additionally, child brides might be permitted in one culture, but would be decried as monstrous in our current culture.

In the last level, the magnitude reaches the proportion of evil. The use and application of this term has always struck me as problematic in the past. While most people can agree that the mass genocide of the Jewish people in World War II is a cultural example of evil, some people try to extend it to countries or people who do not have a worthy magnitude. For example, when President Bush Jr. referred to Iran, Iraq, and North Korea as the Axes of Evil in 2002, this usage seemed more like propaganda than something true or insightful. However, my appreciation of the word has increased as my clinical experience has continued to give me access to the secret thoughts of patients. I would still argue that the use of evil on the political right is too broad, but I am inclined to agree with some patients that what they have done is evil. In work with bad conscience, some patients have confessed that they have tried to break the mind of a romantic partner, or someone with whom they cohabitate, and had a conscious intention to do so. The desire to destroy someone's unified experience of their subjectivity is a demonic magnitude, and as with the other levels, discourse enters here too. In times of war, or in preparation for it, the enemy is demonized, and religious discourse can link abortion to "evil baby murdering."

In summary, the ego drives of the phallic stage have a work group as their object and a parental-substitute who *leads*. Sadism at this level concerns one's image/reputation and group psychology concerns whether the parental-substitute targets, or allows others to target members for slander or disparagement. The phallic stage has an input for decency and the phallic boss, or perhaps a deutero individual who inspires transference, can change the tone away from standards of politeness. At the anal stage the parental-substitute is supposed to *command* and, as Freud (1921) points out in "Group Psychology," this is instrumental for a group to overcome their social anxiety or conscience and let out their uncivilized impulses in war. Hierarchies in organized crime can sometimes mirror army hierarchy, and leadership in both groups allows for members to overcome the anxiety of doing criminal actions.

At the narcissistic stage, the parental-substitute is supposed to *rule*. A king, a secret group like the CIA, or some kind of partly supernatural parental-substitute rules over society and has the power to authorize abject, destructive impulses. However, a violent mob can mirror this power and sanction vicious or "barbaric" behavior upon its perceived enemy. A violent mob or a terrorist group differs from the more organized army or crime family, and the aggression of the former groups is exemplified in both its random outbreaks and random targets. Moreover, this aggression may go further and involve the desecration of the body (ex. lynching). Along with a mob, the deutero phase at this level can be seen in an active-egoist setting up a cult outside of society, or leading a political organization that wants to entirely change society and its ruling ideas. In the cult, for example, the parental-substitute may monstrously sanction having child brides, or a group of "punks" might squat in abandoned buildings and viciously terrorize random people, thus attacking people's feelings of security in being a part of society.[11]

Lastly, at the auto-erotic stage, the parental-substitute appears with the power to *possess* the minds of others. In group psychology, there is the demonization of others in war, which can reach the level of the extermination or wiping away of the enemy as if they never existed. In such cases, there is the sense that without doing so the evil will just grow back or return to infect others. Another example of group psychology at this level is the leader's power of suggestion or the planting or removing of perceptions in the minds of the members. I have worked with patients who undergo "gaslighting" in which their romantic partner is able to cause them to doubt whether she really saw him do what he had done (i.e. saw him kissing another woman in a public place), or whether she had imagined it. At the group level, there seems to be phenomena in which people believe they all witnessed a miraculous event, or, conversely, that something they perceived never occurred at all.[12]

II

There are a few more expressions of the imago that I want to discuss. First, although psychic bisexuality and the horizontal axis will be needed to understand variations, it is possible to present a simple hypothesis regarding the phantastic elements of the Kleinian internal object.

The child is much smaller than its parents, and the greater the magnitude of power of the imago, the greater (i.e. taller and bigger) the parental-substitute will appear in some cases. For example, a classic James Bond movie has the villain who wants to take over the world; the primary villain often has a large henchman underneath him, and these are usually the men with whom Bond must physically contend. Since the main villain is above all humans and does not respect the authority of any society, he is at the narcissistic level. Since his henchman is under him, he would represent the anal level of power. Thus, a large human can express the anal imago. In a fantasy or sci-fi genre, the narcissistic stage imago could be expressed through a creature who is giant, and not merely a large man. The auto-erotic level can include an enormous monster like Godzilla, a mountain that comes alive, or something that is greater than the humanoid (i.e. human-like but exaggerated). Of course, the inverse of this, and representing the self as smaller than the average human is another expression. For example, being the size of an insect, a small animal, or a halfling, dwarf, or hobbit will make a regular human feel much greater. The vampires in *The Lost Boys* are regular-sized, and while this hypothesis has nothing to do with the movie, these ideas are a first step to make sense of some supernatural material.

The second expression of the imago is based upon material from the clinic and concerns the difference between the generations. There is a child-like logic present: just as the parents are more powerful than the child, the parents of one's parents, are more powerful than them. Often grandparents enter the narratives of patients and receive a power and emotional reaction that seems unearned in some cases. This suggests that their appearance is likely part of an imago matrix. Simply, if parents are related to the phallic stage, then grandparents are related to the anal stage, then ancestors are related to the narcissistic stage, and then the gods, supernatural beings, or aliens become the parents in the auto-erotic. This will have some importance when I return for the second data analysis of *The Lost Boys*.

The third expression concerns the complete internalization of the imago that I would like to name the trito phase, in homage to Jones (1933) and following his use of proto and deutero. It is connected to the phenomenon of the full guilt conscience. Freud (1926a) is explicit in his formulation:

> Castration anxiety [that] develops into moral anxiety—social anxiety—and "separation and expulsion from the horde" [in the father complex] only applies to that later portion of the super-ego which has been formed on the basis of social prototypes, not to the nucleus of the super-ego, which corresponds to the introjected parental agency.
>
> *(p. 139)*

As mentioned, social anxiety concerns the ethical life of the community and wanting to have a good reputation. "Originally this sense of guilt was a fear of punishment by the parents, or, more correctly, the fear of losing their love," Freud (1914a) writes, "later the parents are replaced by an indefinite number of fellow-men" (p. 102). However, the father complex concerns the formation of "moral restraint through the process of mastering the Oedipus complex itself, and social feeling through the necessity for overcoming the rivalry that then remained between the members of the younger generation" (Freud, 1923b, p. 37). After the Oedipus complex the active-egoist fears having a reputation of being immoral but will choose immorality if he knows he will not get caught. The individual who traverses the father complex feels equal to peers in the community and will judge himself, even if no one else knows that he has done wrong. Such an individual can also feel guilt about bad intentions that he does not act upon (Freud, 1930, p. 123).

While the social anxiety of the Oedipus complex is based upon the ethical life of one's culture, the guilt of the father complex taps into ideas of fairness and justice that are trans-historical and come from the psychological base of feeling oneself to be equal to others. Freud compares the latter situation to Kant's categorical imperative but with reference to the imago instead of to metaphysical propositions of pure reason (Freud, 1924, p. 167; 1913, p. 22). However, when one considers that there are also prohibitions upon attacking the parental-substitutes upon whom one places the ego ideal, then this also points to morality in the Oedipus complex for those with whom one is intimate or who have power in one's life. Thus, traversing the father complex in the trito phase performs a synthesis of these two oedipal elements. One now has a moral relation to non-intimates who are now felt to be one's equals. In *The Economics of Libido* (2015) I also mention that this traversal involves instinctual renunciation in regards to siblings, as members of one's generation (under the parents). If these impulses are not renounced then one does not properly enter the trito phase and repetitions in the patient's current life can reference love or hate he or she felt for a sibling.

There are several analysts who note a phase of full identification with the imago that may not be reached. For example, there is partial versus full identification with Ives Hendrick (1936, p. 338), establishing the internal good object in Melanie Klein (1940, p. 153), and transmuting internalization in Kohut (1971, pp. 74, 82, 100). Freud (1923b) uses the terms "injunctions and prohibitions" and "social feeling" to impart how this phase will express the feeling of equality with others (p. 37). In common language, it would be apt to contrast the striving for, or possession of happiness in the proto and deutero phases with how the trito phase involves having meaning in one's life. The sense of meaning I have in mind is not some grand existential quest and does not necessarily involve religion or metaphysics, but instead has more to do with how a person seeks to establish fellowship with others. The intellectual meaning that a person gives his fellowship is a secondary elaboration or rationalization, and what is important is the relation of equality to others, no matter what activity they choose to bond over. Lastly, the trito conscience does not mean the oedipal castration complex does not function, but only that the ego or object drive relations to parental-substitutes are offset by the trito conscience. The Oedipus complex comes first and therefore has more power, and one can still be swept up in group psychology.

Notes

1 As mentioned in Chapter 5, people can receive transference based upon the wealth and status of their families and their classes of origin.
2 While many people do not enjoy reading or having to fill internal Space themselves, television, movies, and YouTube clips allow for someone else's internal Space to entertain. Interestingly, these new technologies allow the culture to become functionally schizoid and more detached from community and interactions with others.

3 The synthesizing activity and creativity is something different than just having a good memory, and as Freud (1914a) points out, the lack of the ability to sublimate can lead to an ego injury for those with an ego ideal that demands that they make an ambitious contribution to their field of work. However, without the memory and without the drive to make such a contribution, those with creativity may not reach the standards of good work to have their ideas recognized in their profession.

4 There is more than one type of schizoid, however, and the introduction of psychic bisexuality in the next chapter will give different starting points for the investigation of different behavior at the auto-erotic and other primitive levels.

5 This second example is not an active relation to Time, but I include it to show Time from another angle. Kavaler-Adler (2013) only views time from a persecutory angle while this example shows a depressive one. Moreover, she seems to regard issues with Time in a deficit model instead of conflict: "once a holding mother is internalized—either in infancy, or later in the therapeutic environment with an analyst—the individual can experience a sense of being held by time" (p. 5). As my examples show, it is an intrapsychic conflict that has interpsychic origins. Such people have not always had a persecutory or depressive relation to Time and the deficit model seems prima facie wrong.

6 I have not been consistent with showing how one follows an issue to its end in my clinical examples. Instead, the focus has been to isolate the qualitative level or phenomena that is being investigated in most cases. The primary focus for this book is psychoanalytic theory and the symptom reading and not clinical practice.

7 There are some patients on probation that get filled with massive rage when they are caught violating probation. They will dig their heels in and insist that the positive drug test was wrong, or that their probation officer is the one lying, even when the facts are incontrovertible. To admit that they lied, manipulated, or are "bad" to anal parental-substitutes seems to be connected with a shame so powerful that it must also reference the inability to tolerate pain/frustration at lower levels of development.

8 I will take up the concept of self-sabotage and its ties to other psychoanalytic concepts in the next book.

9 Michael Eigen reports an androgynous combined parent in "The Differentiation of An Androgynous Imago," which indicates an earlier combined parent than "the woman with a penis" of the phallic stage (Eigen, 1975–1976). Additionally, Freud (1918) notes an anal primal scene in the case of the Wolfman concerning the mother being attacked by father (p. 45 fn).

10 I'm open to the idea that the non-universal id impulses that are renounced would have an impact on the body and make physiognomy a potential science. In clinical work, I have often noted bodily similarities between people with similar pathology, but it is not a 100% correlation in my experience. Not everyone with a schizoid personality disorder has the body of an ectomorph, for example. There may be a statistically significant number of them who are ectomorphs, but there is also the issue of having powerful friendships and relations to parental-substitutes that might have helped them to strengthen proto-paternal elements against deutero adaptations. To simply judge someone by their physiognomy is rash, and we have had several decades of analysts like Bion who remind us not to "know" what is wrong with someone because of the arrogance/omniscience in previous generations. Between omniscience and not knowing anything, I hope that psychoanalysts can move forward in a way that is both more modest, but also less ignorant.

11 Group psychology is not merely present in the dynamics of aggression and the lowering of social anxiety. For example, the Republican party in the United States has established a "cult" mentality around climate change, creationism, and the general de-legitimization of academic and scientific consensus. They have convinced their members that certain institutions have become politicized or have a liberal bias and therefore do not have a claim to an objectivity to which we should all defer. As with individual pathology showing how the normal mind works, such pathology in group psychology shows us what is going on in "normal" group psychology. Despite the passion that some liberals have for

climate change, they are mostly basing their concern for global warming on a *social trust* of the academic institutions that say it is a problem. They have not studied the data or the research themselves and some, who are attracted to portraying it as the great problem of the time, do so because of individual pathology that concerns the impersonalized representation of the world or nature from the imago of Space.

12 It is important to understand that this is a relation to the imago of Space and not a complex intellectual idea. In *The Economics of Libido* (2015) I mention anxiety situations of falling forever that come up in patients to similar effect. To have holes in Space itself, as negations of it, does not require that an infant understands concepts in physics. Rather, the reference is how the infant develops ego cognition that allows for a subjective or phenomenological experience of the world and that infant has dynamic relations with the imago involved in these different levels of cognition. In *The Economics of Libido* (2015) I argue that dreams and psychopatholgy require a model like Kant's transcendental idealism in order to be explained. In the next book, I will revisit these arguments and move on to the philosopher Hegel to argue that an even more complicated model is needed.

7

THE SYMPTOM READING (PART 2)

"I could nuke them in their hearts"

Data analysis II

After this long investigation into the oedipal castration complex, and its pre-phallic forms, I was able to return to the film to find another layer of analysis open up. A larger sense of paternity, the mother's phallic image, and regression were now salient to me. I came to see that Sam moves to Santa Carla with his mother after his parents' divorce, and that the vampire metaphor of giving one's blood is not just a representation of Max giving him a new paternity that he rebels against; it is also a representation of the fear of being attached to the paternity of his eccentric grandfather and a similar rivalry with him for who will be "man of the house." Moreover, although choosing an older woman for a day protector does not make sense for a rich and powerful vampire, it does for a grandfather who is old, is not wealthy, and will likely die earlier than his daughter. Additionally, I came to see that the vampires of the symptom plot are linked to another fantasy object: aliens. Sam's grandfather is explicitly linked to aliens. After going through the movie several more times, I began to see that the vampire metaphor is not just linked to paternity but along with aliens it has ties to orphans, stylish punks, and more. I began to tackle more events in the plot that had to receive a new motivation with the excision of the symptom characters.

The symptom characters were initially identified because vampires are not real, and I had the idea to look at the relatively separate plot of Sam as if Michael's plot didn't exist. I began the work of the second data analysis by leaving the particular interactions of the symptom characters and moving to the more general level of the vampire metaphor after I saw the connection between Max and Grandpa at the end of the movie. From their first encounter, Sam's grandfather is linked to vampires. Michael, Sam, and Lucy approach the house and the grandfather is "playing dead" before getting up suddenly and scaring them—an obvious reference to vampires who are dead and supernaturally animated. Additionally, Grandpa scares Sam and Lucy several times more in the film, which links him imagistically to the frightening vampires. Although the lost boys are portrayed as cool by having "hot young stars" Kiefer Sutherland and Jason Patric in the movie (and the movie poster tagline was "Sleep all day. Party all night. Never grow old. Never die. It's fun to be a vampire"), vampires are also represented as foul and bad in the film. They appear young and attractive most of the time, but this is only a ruse that covers their true nature. They are associated with bad breath, foul smells, and flies, and their eyes become animal-like and their faces monstrous in their true form.

Michael, Star, and Laddie fight against their impulses to feed and kill and are never shown as desirous of becoming vampires at all. Sam does not want his brother or Star to become a vampire and the Frog brothers want to kill all vampires and even have to resist killing the good half-vampires. It is only to the extent that the vampires have cool clothes, possessions (David's motorbike, Max's sports car and money), and are linked to music (the giant poster of Jim Morrison in the abandoned hotel where the lost boys live) that they are shown as enviable, or to have something Lucy, Michael, and Sam might like to have. This positive aspect, as well as the bad, murderous aspect, will be discussed later on, but for now I would like to focus on the foul or bad aspect because it is the aspect most linked to the grandfather.

The foul smell of vampires is brought up several times in the film and the grandfather is related to bad smells in several ways. First, Lucy calls him a hippie and by his general appearance the viewer would be led to think he smells. Second, he practices taxidermy and his house has dead animals around, as well as flies; one of the Frog brothers notes the ubiquity of the flies around the undead by suggesting that the two go together like "ham and eggs." The dead animals, along with the embalming fluid used to make them, would no doubt have an unpleasant smell. Third, on his way to a date with the widow Johnson, Grandpa cannot find his aftershave and uses Windex. This causes some revulsion and would associate his character with very strange if not repellant smells. There is also a scene in which Sam wakes up in terror as the camera focuses in on the eyes of one of the stuffed animals and they are linked to the monstrous eyes of the vampires in their bad, foul aspect. Since Sam's grandfather gave them to him, they are linked to his character.

The most important link between Grandpa and vampires is when Sam compares him to an alien or Martian. Structurally both are the same as non-humans and associated with frightening figures in horror movies. Sam mentions this connection three times. The first time he tells his dog, Nanook, that his is a "broken home," that his mother works all day and his brother is asleep all day, and that his grandfather, who practices taxidermy, is "possibly an alien." The second time he asks his brother Michael if he thinks the grandfather is an alien, to which Michael responds, "What would that make Mom?" This shows the worry about how paternity reflects upon the family, and if Lucy is an alien or part alien, then Sam is alien too. The third time is in conversation with the Frog brothers. When Alan Frog asks Sam what he thinks of Santa Clara, Sam sarcastically responds that it is a good place "if you're a Martian." Edgar Frog then adds, "Or a vampire," which sets up the equivalency of the two.

The worry about how the eccentric and alien Grandpa will reflect on Lucy or the boys goes to the heart of the issue. With the departure of Sam's father after the divorce, and the move to Grandpa's house, paternal authority should fall to the eldest male. However, Grandpa lacks Prestige and would be an embarrassing head of the family to a teen like Sam. Before it is revealed that Max is a vampire, he is shown to own "cool" video stores and have lots of money in contrast to the poor, luddite-like grandfather. There is an early scene in which Sam laments about not having a TV at his grandfather's place and that he will no longer know what is "hip" anymore. In contrast, Max has a video store full of TVs. Max also has a dog like Sam, a sports car that Michael likes, and is generally charming.

In regards to phallic Prestige, Max is the opposite of Grandpa and would be a desirable procreator, if Sam did not want to be his own father (and did not transfer the bad phallic mother imago onto him). If Grandpa represents the denigrated paternal imago in these aspects, then, in so far as Max has ties to what is "hip," this likely registers as part of the transference to the remaining half of the paternal imago. Max is an acceptably aged partner for Lucy and, as an adult who owns cool things, this makes him desirable to Lucy from Sam's point of view. Lastly, when Max receives the transference as the bad phallic mother who wants to be his mentor and gives him a phallic image through discipline, this should be contrasted to Lucy receiving the good phallic mother transference. Sam can see himself as man of the house so long as he retains closeness with her on this level. Lucy seems to join her son's disapproval of Grandpa and foster this deutero relation with Sam, in which Grandpa is denigrated. In their first conversation Lucy admonishes her father's current appearance, suggesting that now he dresses like a "hippie," and reminds him that when she was young and dressed in this way, it was he who admonished her. She observes that they have now switched places and are "still out of sync." Later, when Lucy is tucking Sam into bed, Grandpa scares them both producing a woodchuck he has just taxidermied. They both react with "revulsion" to Grandpa's "grotesque" work.

As Sam's symptom, Michael more overtly shows Sam's relation to the denigrated Grandpa.

Early in the film, before Michael attacks Sam, but after he has become a half-vampire, Lucy confronts him about sleeping all day and not doing more for Sam. She laments Sam's constant solitude and we get the sense that he avoids his "Martian" Grandpa. In this respect, Michael is regarded as head of the house by Lucy since she wants him to be the one to deal with Sam, and this is seconded by Max. When Max comes to the house for the date with Lucy he tells Michael that, as he's now "the man of the house" he requires Michael's permission to enter. So far as Michael is excised from the ego plot as a symptom character, I understand that the authority he is conferred reflects the authority that Sam feels in relation to his grandfather. While Sam is shown to reject his grandfather in subtle ways, Michael is quite insolent with him in contrast. Sam is shown as tossing all the stuffed animals his grandfather gives him in the closet and wishing that he would stop giving them to him. In an important scene, Michael both insults his grandfather and, in half-joke form, also shows that he's a potentially dangerous rival. When Grandpa announces that he plans to drop off some taxidermy at the Widow Johnson's, Michael jokes that the stuffed specimen must be Mr. Johnson. Although it feels a little silly to say, "Johnson" was one of the prominent slang words for penis in the 1980s. To recognize this deepens the pun on "Johnson" and "stuffing" by emphasizing Grandpa's castrating aspect. Sam comes to Grandpa's defense and tells Michael that his joke was not funny. This, along with him and Lucy being scared by him numerous times, shows that he is taken seriously at times, and likely oscillates between the denigrated and bad phallic mother transference for Sam.

Grandpa is usually represented as a happy eccentric, but he does remind the boys of his authority. For example, when he first directly addresses Michael and Sam he imperiously yells "rules!" and lets them know what they can and cannot touch in his house, and comes off as pretty serious. There is one scene in particular in which Grandpa's authority comes front and center. When Michael, Sam, and the Frog brothers return with Star and Laddie after taking Grandpa's car they are shown to quietly climb the stairs to avoid detection by him. When he appears he angrily shouts "Michael!" and they all freeze on the staircase. However, he then merely reminds them that there is a "rule" to fill the gas tank when you use the car without permission. The dramatic tension in this scene is what the punishment is to be. When Grandpa reminds them of the "rule," this tone is heavily contrasted with his former tone about rules and the preciousness with which he had treated the car in a previous scene. Grandpa had let Sam know that he does not like the car to be moved and that it is so cherished or treasured, that one is to just sit in it, in the garage. Grandpa's relationship to his car implies a degree of sanctity and non-utilitarian ritual that raises a large specter of potential anger here. Additionally, there is an impression of insult along with the theft when Michael and Sam took Grandpa's 57 Chevy to rescue Star. They ask if they could use it, but peel off before they could hear Grandpa's reply. To excise Michael gets rid of the sense of this act being performed as some emergency, or as exceptional circumstance, and makes Sam's blatant disregard of Grandpa's authority come into focus. Lastly, there is still the question of where Sam and the Frog brothers actually go in this scene, but I will address this later.

When Max reveals himself as head vampire, he becomes part of the symptom plot and a symptom character himself. This means that he must be paired with an ego character. If David is the symptom of Max, and he is killed, then this shows that Max is out of the picture. For example, this might be interpreted as Lucy coming home to see Sam, after another ruined date, but that Max does not come with her. We could imagine that Sam is successful in his defiance and acting out and that Max sees him as a handful and that Lucy is not worth all this trouble. This leaves Grandpa as the remaining authority, and he is linked to Lucy and Max showing up at the house in the script. When Michael, Star, Sam, et al. are standing in the aftermath of the defeat of David, the script calls for a camera shot of Grandpa's truck rumbling down the street and next calls for headlights sweeping across the window. When Sam says "Someone's here," the script creates the expectation that Grandpa was supposed to enter. In the script, the first thing Max says upon arrival is "Where are my boys?" and therefore, I would take him as a symptom character at the moment he arrives.

For Max to become the symptom character of Grandpa gives us an answer as to why Lucy is desired as a "day protector." While it makes little sense for Lucy to be the day protector for the vampires, or the mother who is supposed to control Max's vampire boys, it makes sense that Grandpa would want his daughter to watch over him in his old age. From Sam's vantage point, Grandpa would be sucking/stealing his and Lucy's life by getting them to be caretakers. Lucy would not live long enough to be very valuable to a vampire, but she would live long enough to take care of her father. After David is killed, Michael and the other half-vampires observe that they don't feel any different. Killing the head vampire was supposed to allow them to move back from half-vampire to human, and this indicates that Max felt like the big threat on one level, but on a deeper level Grandpa was the bigger threat.

When Grandpa kills Max, his symptom, the first salient idea is that he kills the bad aspect of himself. In other words, if the vampire-alien metaphor references that authority figures are ethically bad, scary, foul, or weird, then this shows that Grandpa overcomes his denigrated aspect to become the head of the family. Additionally, Michael actually pushes Max into the jeep with the sharpened wood-posts, which implies that he is an accomplice to Grandpa emerging as the paternal authority. Second, after killing Max, Grandpa is shown to have always known about vampires—and thus as wise—even though he is portrayed as foolish, weird, or scary before this. So, where Grandpa would be viewed as wanting to suck the life from Lucy and Sam before, the story ends with the sense that Grandpa should be esteemed for his knowledge and that it is not bad to have affection/loyalty towards him and take care of him. With Grandpa emerging as wise and powerful at the end of the movie, taking care of him might not appear as such a burden and waste. I will have cause to reconsider this below, however.

Now that there is a plausible interpretation of Max becoming a symptom character, and his idiosyncratic desire to enlist Lucy, I want to look at one more aspect of the last scene. As mentioned above, the parental imagos, or the father as head of the family, who possesses the mother, are symbolic of an individual respecting the difference between the generations. Before Grandpa kills Max, Michael was ready to face off with Max and I think it is significant that we regard Grandpa as killing the bad imago aspect of himself (along with Michael's help). This interpretation is tied to the link of the vampire metaphor to another metaphor: that of being a parentless orphan.

When Michael begins "hanging out" with the lost boys in their abandoned hotel lair, they laugh at him for asking where their parents are, and paint him a picture of how they possess "complete freedom." This complete freedom registers strongly at the narcissistic level of authority/Being.

David says that there "are no parents" and "no rules" that no one even knows about the abandoned hotel. In other words, it is outside of the hierarchy in society that is measured by wealth, degrees, and belonging to certain institutions and beneath the imperative of the (phallic and anal) ego ideal to measure oneself in this way. The lost boys still want to impress others on the boardwalk and to be seen as dominant and powerful. So, to be clear, this does not mean that they do not want any recognition/admiration, or lack any connection to others (above seeing them as food). In the script, the leader of a rival gang is described as thinking he is "King of the boardwalk" and this captures the exhibitionism of this kind of relation fairly well.[1]

If we take full vampires as monsters who live outside of society as representing the narcissistic stage, then half vampires like Michael represent the anal stage. The anal level of Being concerns whether or not one is part of civilization and is a non-criminal, tax-paying citizen. Part of the dramatic tension in the film is whether Michael will give in to his impulses "to feed" and kill a human for blood or not. There is a possibility that for Michael to kill Max/Grandpa on his own may register as an attack on the anal parental imago and also mean a regression to the narcissistic level. Vampire status is identified as bad, insofar as the vampires are killers and foul/ugly in true form, and, Michael's resistance to becoming a vampire has two more salient points at the anal level. As mentioned, the badness of the vampires relates to the badness of the anal phallic mother imago. Although we do not see Max or Grandpa murder anyone, the former is revealed as a vampire who must kill others to survive and Michael's joke about Grandpa killing the widow Johnson's husband may be an unconscious expression of this transference. Any rival for the position of "man of the house" would likely receive this transference and be felt to be a bad person whether he has a criminal history or not. Additionally, as mentioned with the alien metaphor, if one is related to a bad person, then this makes one bad too. The second point is that there is evidence that Michael has formed the guilt conscience. This trito phase is dramatized when Michael watches the lost boys kill at the beach and fights his own impulses to kill. The script suggests that the attack is deeply disturbing to him, to the point of nausea, and that when the lost boys call him by name, he must resist a deep urge to join in. Even as half-vampire, Michael's face becomes foul like a full vampire, and though he has not acted on his urges, the intentions alone bother him. I see this as evidence of him having achieved the guilt conscience of the anal trito phase.

Returning to the orphan metaphor, the status of the lost boys as parentless and completely free is paired with their magical abilities. Instead of power that references a field of work, political figures, celebrities, wealth, etc., in society, they have magical powers that show a lack of separation between minds or lack of separation between wish and reality (i.e. defy the laws of physics). For example, Star has some kind of telepathic connection to David and such psychic abilities, along with the vampires flying, show that being a vampire references power in wishing and is the equivalent to hallucinating (narcissistic and auto-erotic stage). In excising these fantastical elements, they can be understood as the danger that a young teen like Sam might become neurotic, or worse, if he does not accept any authority figures.

Although parental imagos still underpin the relations of the primary narcissistic stages, for Sam to murder or do something that will overload the anal stage relations, will lead to a regression in which he will lose drive relations to a human family and society in general. For example, he could become bi-polar and a person who lives day to day and has no future for which to ever plan, or he could retreat into his world of comic books and magical thinking and lose interest in a social life outside of his home.

I will return to the orphan metaphor again later, but the last thing I want to say here about it concerns the phallic stage. Progressively throughout the script Michael is explicitly described as looking more and more like a lost boy. Michael has David's blood in him as a half-vampire and I understand this as Michael accepting David as a parental-substitute at the phallic level. In his behavior, Michael is defiant and attacks with his words and does not seem to care whether Lucy sees him as good, in the sense of being a good older brother to Sam or being polite. These are the hallmarks of the phallic level in contrast to being bad at the anal level as a criminal. This means that the oedipal castration complex is most prominent at the anal stage in this film, although we see the influence of the other stages on Michael's behavior (i.e. the phallic and the vampiric powers of the earlier stages that relate to magical thinking and fantasying).[2]

Above I raised the question of why Sam and the Frogs would steal Grandpa's car to go to the abandoned hotel if Michael, Star, and all the full- and half-vampires of the fantasy plot are excised. Similarly, the excision of the symptom plot points to the importance of the Frog brothers in the final scene before Grandpa and Lucy show up. There are script slips to be analyzed in both events that will help make the latent plot, but, for the moment, I would like to examine the Frogs from their first appearance in the film in order to put together some motivations for the action in these two scenes. Michael finds the lost boys at the boardwalk at the beginning of the film, a scene later paralleled when Sam finds the Frog brothers there too. Although the number of group members is different, three people (i.e. Sam and the two Frog brothers) are still technically a group, and this connection will become important later. The Frog brothers' military style clothing and their claim to be "fighters" for higher principles shows that despite being kids, they would like to be warriors who fight for a cause. This shows the anal stage relation to roles that oppose the dominant culture with a subculture interest. They tell Sam that they are not just comic book store workers, but "fighters" dedicated to higher principles like "truth, justice, and the American way."

Sam's trip with the Frogs is rationalized by Michael wanting to steal Star from David and this hides that Sam is stealing Grandpa's car, in another act of defiance, just as Michael is defying David's claim to Star. Grandpa's prized car can be taken as an equivalent to another man's trophy girlfriend. A certain type of man might not love a woman, but along with his trophies, or other signs of status, he can want to impress others with the "hotness" of his girlfriend. Although such a man may not care deeply for her, he may register humiliation if she cheats on him or is "stolen" by someone else. However, even if Sam steals Grandpa's car in parallel to Michael stealing Star from David, the reason for the trip to the abandoned hotel, specifically, and what goes on there is still a question.

I think a decent answer can be put together from the equivalence set up between the lost boys and the Surf Nazis. At the beginning of the script, the two groups are shown to be two youth gangs who hang out on the boardwalk, and who get into a needless fight. As mentioned, the narcissistic stage castration complex concerns one's relation to society in general.[3] It is easy to imagine that the Surf Nazis might live in a condemned hotel, pay no taxes, and be effectively outside of society like the lost boys. Additionally, it is likely that they would not care about having a career or a good reputation in the community, being at the top of any anal social hierarchies, or obeying the law. Instead, they live outside of human settlements like some mythical monsters that occasionally appear to steal from and terrorize people. One can imagine a group of surfing purists with the view that just living to surf without getting involved in the "rat race" is the ideal life.

Although the lost boys end up killing the Surf Nazis later, if the boys are excised, then we should regard them as alive. A little later in the movie, the Surf Nazis appear in the Frog brother's store and steal some of their comics. In the script this goes further and they destroy the comics, "sprinkle" the remnants over their heads, and walk away laughing. The Frog brothers and Sam are "enraged" and Edgar expresses the wish that they were vampires so he could "nuke them in their hearts," which serves as another link between them and the lost boys. Moreover, there is a rivalry between Sam and the Frog brothers as vampire experts, one that could mirror the stance of Michael to being in the lost boys. Just as Michael begins to look more and more like a lost boy, we see Sam becoming more like a Frog brother and being sucked into their comic book world of vampires. Even though they have commitments to justice and the American way, they also denigrate the anal parental imago. For example, Edgar claims that certain city officials are actually "ghouls" and "werewolves." So, although they want to serve the American way, the Frogs are in a narcissistic position in which they believe that they know "the way" better than the depersonalized anal parental-substitutes. Moreover, in a state of danger in which lawmakers cannot be trusted, there is an implication that their laws do not have to be respected either. Thus, the Frogs accept society (at the narcissistic level), in contrast to the lost boys and Surf Nazis who fully live outside of it, but they feel entitled to break the (anal) laws of civilization. Just as Michael resists David as the bad anal parental imago, the Frogs resist the legitimacy of lawmakers and present Sam with an anal group to join.

Because of the equivalence of the lost boys and Surf Nazis, and the latter's mistreatment of the Frog brothers, it seems plausible that the Surf Nazis might be the target of the Frogs' aggression. Again, it is likely that the Surf Nazis might live like other "punks" do, by squatting in an abandoned building. Therefore, with the excision of the symptom plot, Sam and the Frogs would be going to the hotel lair to attack the Surf Nazis who enraged them, and who sleep during the day because they are up all night partying. As with the lost boys, it likely ends with them getting scared and running away, but there is one loose end. In the movie, as opposed to the script, one of the Frog brothers actually kills a vampire. Murderous impulses to "nuke" them were voiced, but whether we interpret them as doing so or not, does not affect the rest of the latent plot. How would the Surf Nazis know where Sam lives and come after him and the Frogs? There is no evidence that they have talked to Sam or would concern themselves with him at all. It is realistic that the young boys could be paranoid after what they did, and that they might think the Surf Nazis will come after them and find them, but I think the final showdown is really about something else. I will turn to it in a moment.

As mentioned above, there are ties between the Frogs and the lost boys too, as groups that Sam and Michael both find on the boardwalk. Regardless of whether we interpret them as killing a Surf Nazi, they are still militaristic, have a paranoid worldview, take themselves seriously, and are trying to enlist Sam to help them defeat the enemies of America. As mentioned above, Michael and the other half-vampires are never portrayed as desiring to become full vampires. However, Michael registers impulses to want to feed and kill and has to fight them, and Star admits that her desire to kill becomes strong and more difficult to resist each night. In parallel, this can be read as the paranoid Frog brothers exciting Sam's desires to kill or be destructive.[4] If this parallel holds, then this means that Sam would have the same struggle with guilt that Michael does. Moreover, the paranoid worldview of the Frogs, in which evil forces have infiltrated the government and surround their parents' comic book store on the boardwalk, implies a serious commitment for an adherent. In the scene of the hotel raid, the Frogs react to Michael being a half-vampire, and Edgar Frog directly threatens to "stake" Michael if he interferes with their plans. This could be read as a paranoid "with us or against us" mentality that might be used on Sam in the latent plot; the Frogs let Sam know that if he interferes with them attacking the Surf Nazis, they will not hesitate to attack him.

The excision of the symptom plot in the final showdown suggests the conflict is between Sam and the Frogs. Again, it is too far-fetched for the Surf Nazis to know where Sam lives, and there is evidence of an anal group equivalence between the Frogs and the lost boys. Additionally, there is a scene in which the Frogs turn on Laddie, a half-vampire boy who has a close relationship with Star, and who appears on the back of a milk carton as a missing child. The Frogs turning on Laddie is an echo of when they had threatened Michael before the hotel raid, and Michael connects to Sam as his symptom. I would like to spend a bit more time unpacking the reference to Laddie as missing child, or self-chosen orphan, and how his relationship to Star resembles Sam's relationship with Lucy. The idea is that Laddie may be a symptom of Sam here and they turn on Sam as being a "half-member" of their group who does not show full commitment through joining them in murder and/or unquestioning loyalty.

As mentioned above, the "complete freedom" of the lost boys references "no parents" and "no rules" and even the name lost boys references runaway boys or boys who do not have parents (i.e. self-chosen orphans). We have seen how the lost boys' "complete freedom" also registers as a disregard for even the most basic rules of society. Since vampires are fantastical, I compared the threat of becoming a full-vampire to the magical or delusion thinking of someone who is mentally ill. It is possible that there is a connection between this full-vampire state and the orphan metaphor of losing both parents. The previous vampire/alien metaphor references seeing paternal authority in the family as bad/foul, and how Sam does not want to accept it in Max or Grandpa. The metaphor of orphan takes things a step further and references the loss of the maternal connection. In the last part of the movie, Sam has managed to foil Lucy's dates and keep her on his side, but the danger of her choosing Max (i.e. Max finally kisses her when they are on a date) means that Sam could turn his back on her too (and not just paternal figures).

Star and Laddie are half-vampires who are not around their parents, but both show a desire to be with them. Michael has a personal conversation with Star about her estrangement from her parents in a scene in which she pierces his ear. This piercing illustrates how Michael is becoming more like a "lost boy" (i.e. vampire and orphan) and can be taken in parallel to Sam becoming more like the paranoid Frog brothers. In this scene in the script, Star emphasizes that she is not with David romantically and longs for her parents, with whom she used to fight. She implies that she regrets running away as now she "miss[es]" [her] family." Star has run away from her parents but has also resisted committing murder and becoming a full vampire and orphan. Her voicing a longing for a family is further evidence for the tie of how becoming a full lost boy/orphan means no longer wanting parents or missing one's family.

The metaphor of orphan appears very early on in the film, when Lucy meets Max for the first time she first approaches him with a boy who is lost in Max's store. The exchange is quickly interrupted by the boy's young mother, who rushes in to claim him and exclaims how worried she was. The "lost boy" looking for his parents when Max and Lucy are together, is easily interpretable as Sam's desire for a "good" father. I take this as an echo of what I mentioned above, in the representation of Max as being hip and modern. Max works in a cool store with "rock and cartoon images" on the TVs, while Grandpa only reads the TV guide. Again, Sam explicitly laments this situation, noticing that in addition to Grandpa having no TV, there are no malls or Cineplexes in Santa Clara—a place cut off from the rest of civilization. This illustrates the dynamic relation between Max receiving the transference of the bad phallic mother while also receiving the transference of remaining half of the proto-paternal imago. This is the most salient in contrast to Grandpa receiving the transference of the denigrated paternal imago, although we have seen that Grandpa also receives the bad phallic mother transference and that Sam also attacks him as an authority figure too.

Despite this sense that Max might be appealing to Sam on some level and that Sam might want to be in a family with both parents (i.e. proto-oedipal), the orphan metaphor is more powerful as a regression metaphor. So long as Sam keeps ruining his mother's dates and keeps his special relationship with Lucy, he is man of the house, or has the appearance of power in the deutero phase. However, in questioning the legitimacy of the laws in Civilization, going with the Frogs to attack the Surf Nazis, and his reported fears that there are vampires "everywhere," by

Lucy's third date there are grounds for Sam to abandon the anal level of Being. On the third date Sam pleads with his mother to contact the police and the news, and how they will believe her because she is "a mom." As mentioned, she confronts him again about "ruining" another date with Max and he becomes enraged. The orphan metaphor most strongly resonates with Sam's motivation to now push Lucy away too, since she is not on his side here.

The half-vampire boy Laddie, who is close to Star and struggles like her and Michael not to kill, also expresses longing for both his parents. In the script, Laddie tells Star about a recurrent dream in which his father is working in the yard, his red-headed mother brings out drinks and laughs with him, and he plays with the dog. Star tells Laddie that the dream is a memory and makes him promise not to tell David of it, so that he will remain, like her, half-connected to Civilization and the desire for family life. In mentioning the dog and his parents drinking, Laddie gives imagistic links to Sam who has a dog (Nanook) and the date scenes in the movie in which Max and Lucy are shown drinking. This again points to the longing for a father (or both parents) in the orphan metaphor. However, Star and Laddie have a relation that emphasizes a boy with a connection to a maternal figure while the paternal connection is only magical (i.e. David's blood). There is physical closeness in their relationship, Star holds him and hugs him, and when Michael visited Star the script indicates that he noticed Laddie sleeping "nearby." This resembles Sam getting into bed with Lucy and resting with her. Similarly, Star rescues Laddie from David's influence, and Lucy leaves her dates with Max to come and save Sam. These parallels between Sam/Lucy and Laddie/Star suggest that we should see Laddie as a symptom of Sam in the final showdown.

When the Frog brothers plot to turn on the half-vampires, and Laddie emerges to attack them, Star runs to him and hugs him and he reverts from his monstrous vampire form back to normal. In parallel, this means a latent reading of Sam wanting to kill the Frogs after hearing them plot on him for not fully committing to their authority. However, as Star appears to calm Laddie down, Sam's deutero phase connection to Lucy proves strong enough to calm him down. This intrapsychic relation in Sam, as we know, is also paralleled by an interpsychic one in which Lucy leaves the date with Max to come home and presumably try to calm Sam as she had done before. However, before Lucy and Grandpa return to the house, and after Laddie's near attack on the Frogs, there is Michael's fight with David, which now must be re-evaluated.

Before Lucy and Grandpa return, Sam presumably has the worry that he is still going to lose Lucy to Max. At the same time, the latent plot suggests he heard the Frogs plotting against him. There is evidence that Sam must wrestle with the idea of Max winning over Lucy and with his conscience in regards to fully joining the Frogs' paranoid worldview. As mentioned above, since Max enters the final scene as a symptom character (i.e. his first line is to ask where his boys are), and Grandpa's headlights flash on the window in the script, we should interpret that Lucy leaves Max and Grandpa coincidentally comes home just a little later. Although the interpretation of Grandpa killing the denigrated and bad phallic mother relation in himself is likely still applicable, Max should also be regarded as a symptom of whoever Sam experiences as the leader between the two Frog brothers. Thus, when Grandpa shows up to kill Max, this is best interpreted as him establishing his authority over the Frogs. Presumably, Sam first successfully fights his impulses to murder them, but still ends up fighting one of the Frogs who are still trying to get him to commit to their cause. Sam wins the fight and establishes that he will not enlist with them. However, the Frogs still claim that he is already one of them, which references how Michael's defeat of David does not change the half-vampires back to humans, and that Sam still lacks good paternity in Grandpa and fears having him or Max take on this role. Presumably, Sam and the Frogs had trashed the house in their fight, and in their paranoia about retaliation from the Surf Nazis. Then, an angry Grandpa returns home, kicks out the Frogs, and forbids Sam to talk to them. Since vampires do not exist, this effectively solves the "vampire problem" by getting rid of the Frog brothers who have been peddling their horror comics and paranoid thoughts to Sam.

I have argued that the anal castration complex is the dominant superego conflict and the threat of further regression looms in the film. Furthermore, I have interpreted that David's blood in Michael and the latter's irresponsible and impolite behavior indicate acceptance of the bad parental imago on the phallic level. I would like to also add the script directions, in a scene in which Star pierces his ear, that Michael begins to look more like a lost boy "every minute," as an expression of this phallic acceptance. Additionally, this parallel holds with Sam, who prepared for the final showdown with the Frogs, and also begins to adopt their style. However, the psychoanalytic theory in the last two sections also indicates that this may be the expression of something else as well.

We have seen that the splitting of the paternal imago goes along with creation of the phallic mother's phallic image along with the denigration of one half of the paternal imago. In the script there is an additional scene that suggested the importance of Lucy giving Sam a phallic image, as opposed to just the threat of Max trying to give Sam his image of a "good boy." The scene takes place after the heroes rescue Star and Laddie and leave the lost boys' lair, and are returning home in Grandpa's car. A "cop" pulls them over and they manage to evade any issues by pretending to be a "punk" band. One would think that this would work, in part, because Michael has adopted the "punk" style of the lost boys' clothes, but this is also a comment on Sam and the Frogs since they are in the vehicle too. Additionally, earlier in the film, the script also directs for Sam to make his hair into "punkish styles" with soap while he is in the bathtub, which establishes some interest in this style for Sam too.

We have already seen how Lucy shows some antipathy for her father's style and feels out of sync with him, but along with this Lucy shows attraction to the "hip" style of counter-culture youth. Early in the movie, Lucy runs into the lost boys at Max's video store and tells Max that they are like her when she was younger but "dress better." She associates them to her own "hippie" adolescence, and there is a further connection of the lost boys to the counter-culture of Lucy's youth in that they have a giant poster of Jim Morrison in their lair. Interestingly, Jason Patric, who plays Michael, also strongly resembles Jim Morrison and the movie prominently features contemporary music throughout, with one band doing a cover of a Doors song. Since Sam wants to watch MTV and know what is "hip," this connection with the lost boys referencing Lucy's taste shows another positive aspect of the vampire metaphor. With the explicit connection between this positive aspect and the denigrated aspect of Grandpa, it is a good candidate for being Lucy's phallic image. Thus, as Michael begins to look more and more like a lost boy, his defiance to paternal figures is balanced with becoming more like what his maternal figure wants. As mentioned, to the extent that the Frogs are accepted as part of the punk band in the car then this plays in with Lucy's phallic image. However, it is also possible that part of Sam's resistance to joining the Frogs is not just his moral prohibitions, but his interest in the stylish aspects of society that the Frogs don't appreciate in their military mentality.

There are two last theoretical issues regarding the analysis of the vampire metaphor through the different levels of Being. The first is that although regression from the anal to the narcissistic level takes one to wishful, magical power instead of socially recognized power, this does not mean that group psychology does not function any longer. Again, David and his lost boys exist outside of society in an abandoned hotel, without paying taxes, and with no interest in money, status, etc. They share identity with the more realistic Surf Nazis and similar antisocial groups or mobs who commit monstrous crimes or terrorize random people who are a part of society. Additionally, these groups also share a functional parallel with some religious cults and communes in which members "live off the grid" and often have antagonistic views with how humanity is corrupt, evil, ignorant, and misguided, and often times worthy of destruction. The Frogs seem to have the nascent ideology at this level because of the depth of their paranoia, but also function at the anal level and show a basic acceptance of "America." David is only represented as being in love with his own freedom and shows no bigger agenda or worldview. As a vampire, he is already immortal and need not fight for his own individual recognition by humanity, nor for the recognition of the supremacy of the American way over all other ways.

The second issue concerns the importance of oral symbols in the film. As I showed in Chapter 1, symbols, bodily zones, and id impulses have become a very important part of my clinical work. The problem is that it is difficult to align them with a specific stage and phase and that it is clear that many, if not all, of the zones are related to more than one impulse (i.e. oral cannibalism, oral swallowing whole, oral biting with fangs or the two front teeth, etc.). Because of the confluence of different levels of Being in multiple transferences to one person, it is difficult to know which stage/phase is in operation in the clinic. Although it is not much easier when working with these symbols in a film, this work has to begin, and with enough data from different films, there will be a way to find similarities and organize it. I would like to give a first attempt here, while also letting my reader know that much more organized work will follow in the next book.

In the last two chapters I showed how the auto-erotic stage aligns with Space and Freud's concept of the mnemic trace. I articulated this as the idea that one's own fantasy life (i.e. internal Space) can compete with the things that exist in the external world (external Space) so that hallucinations can be explained. In *The Lost Boys*, vampiric powers like flying register like hallucinations at the auto-erotic level, in contrast to the unobservable psychic powers of the narcissistic stage like telepathy, 'the power of positive thinking,' and practice like Reiki. Freud (1930) acknowledges the breast as part of the first stage of the reality principle in which the infant needs to discern between hallucinating the breast and the real breast that actually gives nourishment/milk (pp. 66–67). Cartons, both food and milk cartons, show this link between nourishment and hallucination in the film. Early in the movie, Michel attempts to eat Chinese food from cartons (the word is in the script) but David changes the food to maggots and worms, to which Michael reacts with revulsion and disgust. This suggests that David also registers as a God-like auto-erotic parental-substitute because he controls Michael's perceptions. After Michael drinks David's blood, he goes to drink milk from the carton in the fridge at Grandpa's, but he "buckles over in pain," drops the carton, and it "bursts open," as directed in the script. Lucy ends up cleaning up the mess later and the carton also becomes significant because it has Laddie's picture and his status as lost or missing. Orality that is connected to hunger, which is also connected to hallucinations, someone who controls one's perceptions, to revulsion and disgust, as well as a breast bursting open are all tied together here.

Since Michael's body cannot accept the good milk or nourishment, it seems like he is tempted, like the lost boys, to get the essence or life force from the bodies of others in their blood. One's experience of one's body in physical Space, by reciprocity, also points to the existence of the bodies of others in external Space. If one's body is empty and hungry, then a reciprocal phantasy is that another body is full and bountiful. I have had some depressed patients who have fantasied an apple or round, breast-like object and in the fantasy they pierce its skin with their front teeth and this puncture is the cause of the apple beginning to wither away. They are in PI with the breast and describe fantasies in which their bodies are withering away, and when their skin eventually withers down to the bone, then they often imagine that their bones turns to dust that is blown away in the wind. Additionally, with some of them there is sometimes a fantasy of paradise or heaven in which every comfort and need is present ("a land of milk and honey"). In the relation to the imago of Space there is also a potential fantasy of not a body but a place of fullness in which ideal symbiosis can exist. Although the connections between the imago of Space, God, and orality is easy enough to see, the different libidinal positions of psychic bisexuality on the horizontal axis, the different phases in the stage, and the defenses of PI all still have to be sorted. Again, I hope to give my reader more in the next book.

Lastly, the latent story that emerges from the symptom reading would go something like this: a boy and his mother move in with his grandfather after his parents' divorce. The departure of his father, along with the unsuitability of his eccentric grandfather as a father figure, means that the boy wants to be his own father: the "man of the house." The boy fears both that his grandfather will reflect badly on his image, and also that his mother will have to become a caretaker for him and lose her own vitality. However, his mother soon secures a job and her new boss asks her on a date and this new threat comes much more into the foreground. The boss is seen as possessing the charm, modernity, and money that the boy's grandfather lacks, but at the same time the boy does not want to lose his feeling of authority in the house. Moreover, the boy senses that the man would like to change him and feels that he is bad in some kind of way, and letting him close would make him bad too. The boy tries to ruin their dates by making up fantastic stories about vampires. He also manipulates his mother's concern by getting her to let him sleep in her bed with him. This lets him feel like he is still the man in her life. The boy, in his frustration at the rivalry for his mother begins to have murderous and criminal impulses arising.

The boy specifically chose vampire stories to tell his mother because he had earlier met two brothers on the boardwalk of the new city whose parents own a comic book store. They had given him a few comics and he began to identify with them in some ways. These boys try to get him to join them as fighters for justice and the American way, and offer the boy a paranoid view of the world. They feed into his worries about his mother's suitor being immoral in some way, and the boy gets their help to ruin one of his mother's dates. Later, the boys are antagonized by a local gang who destroys some merchandise at their (parents') store, and in their rage the boys decide to exact justice. They get the boy to come with them to attack the gang in the abandoned hotel in which they live, and express that they are either with them or against them. The boy resists taking part in this and the fighters for justice get scared of the resistance that the gang gives them. They return to the boy's home, with the initial fear that the gang members will retaliate, but the true fight occurs when the boy overhears the brothers' distrust of him and that they will turn on the boy after the fight with the gang. This leads to the boy standing up for himself and he gets into a fight with one of the brothers and the house is trashed.

The boy's status as a part of the brothers' paranoid group and his status as man of the house come to a head at this point. His mother had chosen to go on her third date with her boss and had not listened to her son's excuses, fears, or lies to ruin it for her. The boy's conscience will not allow him to give in to his antisocial impulses and he knows that the brothers will not accept him if he is not as fully committed as they are. Ultimately, guilt gets the best of the boy's mother and she cancels the date to check on her son and her boss loses interest in seeing this dysfunctional dynamic between the two of them. First the boy's mother returns home and shortly afterwards his grandfather ends up returning home and scares the brothers off. In doing this, the boy overcomes his feeling that his grandfather is weird and interested in sucking the life out of him and his mother by making them his caretakers. He accepts his grandfather as head of the family and possibly escapes regressing, defending against his impulses, and becoming mentally ill or identifying with his aggressors in a paranoid view of the world.

Notes

1 There is a little evidence for the connection of the exhibitionism of the lost boys and Sam's character. Although it seems strange to imagine Sam as a "tough guy" who wants to bully others on the boardwalk, he "shows off" when he first meets the Frog brothers and explains to them how they have wrongly arranged their comics. After Sam impresses them with his comic book knowledge, Edgar Frog asks him if he is from "Kryton," referencing Sam being an alien from another planet and tying him to the vampire/alien metaphor. However, instead of its bad aspect as subhuman, this seems to reference it in a superhuman, or more powerful than human way. This powerful aspect of the alien/vampire metaphor is discernable, but, again, the bad foul aspect is much stronger and we don't see much evidence for the longing for this power in Michael or Sam.

2 The correlation of the anal stage imago with grandparents is seen in Grandpa emerging as the ego character for Max entering the symptom plot.

3 The vampire metaphor also includes the idea that people who live like the lost boys and Surf Nazis are functionally "immortal." Instead of having to achieve this through work or recognized social authority or power, they are above humanity, although not completely over it. As mentioned in the last section, the narcissistic stage concerns being in sync with humanity vs. being in one's own Time in different types of psychopathology. In *The Economics of Libido* (2015), I draw attention to movies like *Highlander* (1987) in which immortals live among normal people. The narcissistic stage seems to have an element in which these immortals must battle with others because "there can only be one." This can be illustrated in a more covert way with the idea that someone who acts, or comports himself, like he is king, is going to annoy others. The leader of the Surf Nazis, Greg, is described by the script as thinking that he is "king of the boardwalk." To say someone thinks he is "king" when there is no scepter, crown, or sign, means that the assessment is made through how he treats others and how he carries himself. To walk around like one "owns the place" and to get in the way of others, or to walk with lordly affectation—like one is incredibly tough or staring others down, for example—is often an offense to the pride of other active-egoists. Whether it is treating others poorly or just the non-verbals, such people can give off the impression of severe grandiosity. In the last section I linked such grandiosity to being the maternal imago in the proto relation (i.e. in projective identification). In the deutero relation, one has a strong self-confidence, like one is a prince or has something special, which would make the king have an interest in them. While the grandiose person would feel that their thoughts, or beauty, or talents, etc. are worth as much as a king's or immortal's, the deutero individual at this stage is not as grandiose as this.

4 Additionally, it is also possible that their cause of "truth, justice, and the American way" can be interpreted as a longing for the good aspect of a paternal figure, so that the proto-paternal imago is relevant here and not just the bad deutero aspects. In the film, the Frog brothers' parents are portrayed as hippies that are asleep in the comic book store. This implies that their ideology doesn't come from their parents and also that they may be functionally orphans with no rules or expectations on them. If their ideology does not come from their parents it increases the sense of it as a parental function that gives them guidance and rules that they view as good, and that Sam can similarly have this relation to it.

CONCLUSION

In the analysis of *The Lost Boys* (1987) I stumbled upon the idea of creating a latent plot through an exploration of doubling within the film. The construction of the latent plot in the symptom reading goes beyond building insight into a character or author. It works with the entire story: making sense of idiosyncratic elements of the manifest plot and putting constraints on doubling in the service of the latent plot. Surveying the analysis there are six steps to the procedure that I would like to formalize.

Throughout all of these steps, one will often find small textual clues that will either be needed to build meaning or can be used to corroborate the links between characters that one has already established. I have taken to calling them *script slips*. They follow principles of condensation, displacement, work with symbols, and work with a rebus or other forms of wordplay. These are found in Freud's "Interpretation of Dreams" (1900) and, of course, are created through a patient's associations to manifest content. I did not ask the scriptwriter, or someone involved in making the film, to associate to content in the film. However, we are not concerned with the personal unconscious of these people and how some of the material might associate to traumatic or repressed memories of their past. Instead, we are concerned with the objective aspects that create trans-historical symbols and are involved in some forms of word play, and which the analyst is able to guess, at times, in work with a patient. It is very thin evidence to hang an interpretation on one association, and my reader will find that these script slips are only treated as the icing and not the cake itself in most cases. In the places in which the script slips are used to provide the main evidence for an interpretation, I have made sure to show that there are several of them, or find other evidence to corroborate the direction to which they point.

The first step is to examine the manifest plot for troubling or idiosyncratic plot points, to find what I will call the *red thread* in homage to Wilhelm Reich. David is fixated on getting Michael to join him and become a full-vampire and later we find out that this was Max's command and part of his plan to get to Lucy through her sons. Max had the idea that if he got Lucy to join him that she would help him to better control the other lost boys (or become a protector for him during the day, in the script). It is difficult to see why the lost boys would somehow listen to a random woman and begin behaving better. If Lucy is supposed to be special and have rare powers of love and kindness that would win them over, it is hard to see how she could be OK with the killing that the vampires do. As an older woman without any skill in combat it does not make sense to have her as a day protector. Lastly, any cover she might provide for Max, such as making him appear as a family man does not seem necessary and would not last long before Lucy ages.

The second procedure is to isolate the symptom character(s). In the literature review we saw several ways to determine a latent double. The primary idea was moral complementarity in which the moral goodness might necessitate a double to express moral badness (Rogers). Another approach was seeking manifest textual evidence of two characters having a special tie or metaphysical bond (Keppler). Another was to take an idiosyncratic reaction of one character, which was not motivated in the plot, and look for the textual evidence that the reaction better fits another character (Freud). Another approach is to examine two subplots for latent textual relations so that one of them will help explain the idiosyncratic behavior in another (Tarratt). Lastly, there is the general sentiment of shared identity that is expressed in two different ways. First, it can come from family, shared profession, shared experiences, shared social status, etc., and two characters generally being like one another. Second, there is shared identity that comes from structural consideration of two characters being together at the beginning or end of the film, or at some pivotal point in the plot (Rogers).

To these various forms of identifying a latent double, I would add the further criteria of the would-be double appearing as wish fulfillment. By this I mean that in cases in which there is a supernatural or fantastical character that does not exist in the real world (i.e. vampire, demon, wizard, etc.), this character, or characters, represents wishful thinking. However, in cases in which there is not a fantastical character there are still characters who are very improbable, although they are human. For example, for one character to be shipwrecked on a desert island and find another person already there with whom he falls in love, is far-fetched. Similarly, for a character who lives a mundane life in the suburbs to also possess a secret life in which he or she is a CIA agent is equally improbable and also contains a fantastical/wish fulfillment quality.

In *The Lost Boys*, I established the double by the fantastical nature of vampires. Michael, the older brother, was turned into a half-vampire by David, the leader of the lost boys. Michael was involved in his own subplot with vampires, and though Sam entered the subplot later, excising Michael as the double, along with all the other vampire elements with which he was involved, was straightforward. This left the more realistic, ego plot of Sam dealing with his mother going out on dates with her boss.

The third procedure is to isolate the inter-relation(s) of the symptom character(s) in order to transcribe them to the ego character(s). As mentioned in the introduction, the symptom reading is only applying what we see in the manifest plots of some texts to texts that do not have a surprise ending. For example, at the end of Alfred Hitchcock's *Psycho* (1960) we find that Norman Bates had been impersonating his dead mother all along and that he was responsible for the murders. After identifying the double, there is a dialectical procedure of identifying a double's actions, or behavior in a triangle, and then finding the moments in which the inter-relations can be attributed to the primary, or *ego character*.

Michael has two major relations to Star and David. Michael falls in love with Star and this is triangulated with David. Star is a half-vampire, like Michael, and belongs to David through this tie and Michael attempts to steal her away from him. The other major relation is David's obsessive attempts to recruit Michael into the vampire group and Michael's continued resistance. Even after Michael (and his group) destroyed the other lost boys, David still asks Michael to join him. David's special interest in Michael and the latter feeling like he is an equal of David while also seeing him as morally bad, characterizes the relation.

We see these two relations transcribed to Sam at the moments in which Sam references Michael in his plot. This transcription occurs in the moment when Sam's mother, Lucy, is on dates with Max, her boss, and Sam tells his mother that Michael, or vampires in general, are threatening him. On one hand, Sam is stealing his mother away from an acceptable adult partner (i.e. the special tie that Star has with David). On the other hand, we saw that the subtext showed that Max has a special interest in marrying Lucy in order to be a father to Sam, and become his mentor. Sam testing Max to see if he is a vampire, along with sabotaging the dates, shows how Sam defies the mentoring relationship that Max wants. Thus, moments that reference the symptom character or plot, or moments in which the symptom character impinges on the relations of the ego character to others, serve as a rationalization for the moments in which the inter-relations that that symptom character expresses are enacted by the ego character.

The fourth procedure follows the recognition that Lucy's boyfriend and boss, Max, is revealed as the head vampire at the end of the film, and therefore must become a symptom character himself.

This is the *navel* of the symptom reading and should be approached in two different ways. First, the second-wave symptom character requires the same treatment laid out in the third step. Second, in the excision of the symptom character(s), aspects of the manifest plot are often left hanging and need to be explained. For example, if the ego character was going to see the symptom character at place X in the film, and the symptom character is excised, then why would the ego character still go there? An important difference between the first and second-wave symptom characters is that the former should be regarded as never having existed in the latent plot, while the latter are excised only when they become symptom characters.

By examining the script slips that created ambiguity about whether Grandpa was going to arrive after Michael defeated David, I argued for interpreting Max as becoming the symptom of Grandpa. Additionally, without Michael and the lost boys, I had to make sense of why Sam and the Frog brothers wanted to steal Grandpa's car and go to the abandoned hotel. This was interpreted as partly relating to Grandpa receiving the transference that Max/David received and how Sam stealing Grandpa's prized car was comparable to Michael stealing Star away from David. As for the destination of the hotel, a plausible case was made that the Frogs might have wanted to seek revenge on the Surf Nazis for terrorizing the boardwalk and stealing from their comic store. There were some clues to shared identity between the Surf Nazis and the lost boys to be found in the original film script to justify this.

The fifth step in the procedure is to take the second-wave symptom character and do two things. First, one builds a case for how the red thread of step 1 receives a more realistic motivation from the excision of the second-wave symptom character. Second, beyond the specific inter-relations of a symptom character, his, her, or its excision point to a larger category of identity that should be dissected into different qualities; these qualities provide more insight into the ego character(s) in the film.

Instead of Max wanting Lucy to somehow help him control the lost boys, the vampire metaphor indicates that from Sam's point of view, Grandpa is old, weird, scary, and disgusting. Grandpa could want to "suck the life out" of his mother by having her take care of him. We also saw how the final showdown at Grandpa's house was most plausibly interpreted as Sam getting into a fight with the Frog brothers who turned on him in the latent plot, just as they aggressed Laddie, the half vampire boy, in the manifest plot. The connection between Laddie and Sam was made through the analysis of the orphan aspect of the vampire metaphor and similarities between Star rescuing Laddie and Lucy coming to rescue Sam were found.

The last step is to write up the whole latent plot. After all this work of transcription and identifying important metaphors, writing up a latent plot to highlight the most important material is very satisfying. This summary shows the "real (hidden)" and more neurotic meaning of the text that was covered up by the wish-fulfilling symptom characters.

In summary:

1. Identify the *red thread*, or the troubling or idiosyncratic plot point in the manifest plot by examining differences of opinion in the criticism or by arguing for the ill-logic of a plot point because of it being irrational or out of character.
2. Identify the first-wave symptom and ego character(s).
3. Show the symptom character's inter-relations and find the moments that they can be transcribed to the ego character, as if the symptom character never existed.
4. Find the *navel* of the symptom plot, which introduces second-wave symptom and ego characters and look for events that require motivation with the first-wave symptom character being excised. Identify the second-wave symptom and ego characters as was done in step 1. Identify the motivations for events in the manifest plot that are left hanging by the excision of the symptom characters through following textual clues.

5 Make an argument for how the red thread of step 1 gets a more sensible motivation from the second-wave ego character(s). More broadly examine the symptom character metaphor and its ties to other metaphors or themes in the text in order to understand the navel of the symptom reading.
6 Write up a summary of the new latent plot so that the most important themes can be emphasized and the full neurotic glory of the text, previously hidden under wish fulfillment, can be exhibited.

Absent from these steps is any kind of investigation into the psychoanalytic literature, aside from familiarity with the techniques of dream interpretation. I would not expect the non-clinician to do any more than to provide a latent reading that follows the six steps. Such a reading, on its own, is valuable because it will contribute to the data that will require meta-analyses down the road and show the unconscious repetitions that have remained under-theorized in psychoanalysis.

Lastly, after viewing *The Lost Boys*, I formulated a hypothesis about the "objective code" of the symptom reading that I mentioned in the introduction. Different genres show different motivational structures in their characters and these issues from the motivational structures in the filmmakers and resonate with the ones in the audience members. The filmmakers identify with the central character(s) they (re-)write, and when their complexes, which are tied to anxiety, unpleasure, or superego tensions come up in relation to the motivations given to the character, they externalize them onto a fantasy or symptom character. In this way, the enjoyment of the ego or reality-based character is not reduced by anxiety, what a person thinks they should be, or any unconscious need for punishment (i.e. superego). As mentioned, I found that Robert Rogers (1970) had already formulated this hypothesis and the first symptom reading does not seem to disprove or challenge it. I will continue to evaluate it in the next book.

I would like to make one further comment about the interpretation of *The Lost Boys*. It concerns certain symbols and phantasies in the movie. Where Freud's genius gave us the centrality of the Oedipus complex and the superego to understand character, Klein's genius gives us fuller appreciation of the phantasy and id impulses that underpin it. In the scene entitled "One Big Coffin," in which Sam, Michael, and the Frogs go to the hotel lair to steal away Star, they come upon the lost boys hanging upside down in a cave. Klein (1975) writes of a patient who had "phantasies about his mother's 'inside' as a place of danger. For he felt he had attacked and injured the imaginary babies inside his mother's body and they had become his enemies" (p. 13). Klein (1940) also discusses this phantasy, or variations of it, in other places, and the scene in the film produced an uncanny resonance (p. 136; 1935, p. 166).

Part of the symptom reading's ability to generate data comes from matching the level of Being in the superego with different id drives, erotogenic zones, or specific phantasies like this one. However, as we have seen, every level of superego development is represented in the movie in some way, and the level the phantasy should be assigned to is unclear. Furthermore, in the next book I will go into much more detail about the active/passive binary of psychic bisexuality and expand it into four distinct libidinal positions. This means that every superego stage can be broken down into three phases and that each phase can conceivably be expressed in four different libidinal positions. Additionally, I have mentioned that this full economics of libido—with a vertical and horizontal axis—must also be contrasted to an economics of punishment and anxiety conversion.

The psychoanalytic model of mind that I will continue to construct is complex, and because of the empathy required, there will be many who resist it. They will not have the feeling for it, and will prefer to hide in the infinite possibilities of postmodernism or an atomistic rational chooser model. Even those who have a feeling for it will be resistant because of the ethical allegiances they have formed in identity politics. They may have commitments to the importance of gender roles, for example, and be disposed to deny any input from individual psychology. I do not expect people to take seriously anything for which evidence is not provided. This is undoubtedly a grand project that attempts to classify erotogenic zones, phantasies, id drives, and symbols, with the levels of superego development, which in turn all link to the character traits displayed in the phenomenology of common language. There are many who will say that such a model is immodest, but one should not fail to see that they have also made a Prestige-granting industry out of their humility.

BIBLIOGRAPHY

Allen, R. (1999). *Psychoanalytic Film Theory: A Companion to Film Theory* (Toby Miller and Robert Stam, Eds.). Malden, MA: Blackwell.

Beres, D. (1958). Viscissitudes of Superego Functions and Superego Precursors in Childhood. *Psychoanalytic Study of the Child*, 13: 324–351.

Bergler, E. (1938). Preliminary Phases of the Masculine Beating Fantasy. *Psychoanalytic Quarterly*, 7: 514–536.

Bernhard, H. (Producer) & Schumacher, J. (Director). (1987). *The Lost Boys* [Motion Picture]. USA: Warner Bros.

Bieber, I. et al. (1962). *Homosexuality: A Psychoanalytic Study*. New York: Basic Books.

Bion, W.R. (1959). Attacks on Linking. *International Journal of Psychoanalysis*, 40: 308–315.

Blum, J. (1988). *Transcending Gender: The Male/Female Double in Women's Fiction*. Rochester, NY: University of Rochester Press.

Brontë, C. (1847/1984). *Jane Eyre* (Q.D. Leavis, Ed.). London: Penguin.

Brunswick, R.M. (1940). The Preoedipal Phase of the Libido Development. *Psychoanalytic Quarterly*, 9: 293–319.

Byrne, R. (2008). *The Secret*. New York: Simon & Schuster.

Chasseguet-Smirgel, J. (1976a). Freud and Female Sexuality: The Consideration of Some Blind Spots in the Exploration of the "Dark Continent." *International Journal of Psychoanalysis*, 57: 275–286.

Chasseguet-Smirgel, J. (1976b). Some Thoughts on the Ego Ideal: A Contribution to the Study of the "Illness of Ideality." *Psychoanalysis Quarterly*, 45: 345–373.

Davis, D. (2005). Echo in the Darkness. *Psychoanalytic Review*, 92(1): 137–151.

Doane, M.A. (1991). Dark Continents: Epistemologies of Racial and Sexual Difference in Psychoanalysis and the Cinema. In M.A. Doane, *Femmes Fatales: Feminism, Film Theory, Psychoanalysis*, 209–248. London: Routledge.

Dolar, M. (1991). "I Shall Be with You on Your Wedding-Night": Lacan and the Uncanny. *Rendering the Real*, 58: 5–23.

Eder, D.L. (1978). The Idea of the Double. *Psychoanalytic Review*, 65(4): 579–614.

Edgcumbe, R. & Burgner, M. (1975). The Phallic-Narcissistic Phase: A Differentiation Between Preoedipal and Oedipal Aspects of Phallic Development. *Psychoanalytic Study of the Child*, 30: 161–180.

Eigen, M. (1975–1976). The Differentiation of an Androgynous Imago. *Psychoanalytic Review*, 62(4): 601–613.
Eigen, M. (1977). On Breathing and Identity. *Journal of Humanistic Psychology*, 17(3): 35–39.
Eigen, M. (1983). On Time and Dreams. *Psychoanalytic Review*, 70: 211–220.
Eigen, M. (1986). *The Psychotic Core*. London: Karnac Books.
Eigen, M. (1993). *The Electrified Tightrope* (A. Phillips, Ed.). Northvale, NJ: Aronson.
Eigen, M. (1995). Psychic Deadness: Freud. *Contemporary Psychoanalysis*, 31: 277.
Eigen, M. (2004). *Psychic Deadness*. London: Karnac Books.
Eigen, M. (2016). Image, Fullness, Void. *Psychoanalytic Inquiry*, 36(8): 613–619.
Elias, N. (1994). *The Civilizing Process*. Malden, MA: Blackwell.
Erikson, E. (1963). *Childhood and Society*. New York: W.W. Norton.
Fairbairn, W.D. (1952). *Psychoanalytic Studies of the Personality*. London: Tavistock Publications.
Fenichel, O. (1949). The Symbolic Equation: Girl = Phallus. *Psychoanalytic Quarterly*, 18: 303–324.
Ferenczi, S. (1952). First Contributions to Psycho-Analysis. *International Psychoanalytical Library*, 45: 1–331.
Forman, M. (1976). Narcissistic Personality Disorder as a Regression to a Preoedipal Phase of Phallic Narcissism. *Hillside Journal of Clinical Psychiatry*, 3(1): 45–59.
Freud, S. (1900). The Interpretation of Dreams. In J. Strachey (Ed.), *The Standard Edition of the Complete Psychological Works of Sigmund Freud, Volume IV (1900): The Interpretation of Dreams (First Part)*, ix–627. London: Hogarth.
Freud, S. (1905). Three Essays on the Theory of Sexuality. In J. Strachey (Ed.), *The Standard Edition of the Complete Psychological Works of Sigmund Freud, Volume VII (1901–1905): A Case of Hysteria: Three Essays on Sexuality and Other Works*, 123–246. London: Hogarth.
Freud, S. (1907). Obsessive Actions and Religious Practices. In J. Strachey (Ed.), *The Standard Edition of the Complete Psychological Works of Sigmund Freud, Volume IX (1906–1908): Jensen's "Gradiva" and Other Works*, 115–128. London: Hogarth.
Freud, S. (1908). "Civilized" Sexual Morality and Modern Nervous Illness. In J. Strachey (Ed.), *The Standard Edition of the Complete Psychological Works of Sigmund Freud, Volume IX (1906–1908): Jensen's "Gradiva" and Other Works*, 177–204. London: Hogarth.
Freud, S. (1909a). Analysis of a Phobia in a Five-Year-Old Boy. In J. Strachey (Ed.), *The Standard Edition of the Complete Psychological Works of Sigmund Freud, Volume X (1909): Two Case Histories ("Little Hans" and the "Rat Man")*, 1–150. London: Hogarth.
Freud, S. (1909b). Notes Upon a Case of Obsessional Neurosis. In J. Strachey (Ed.), *The Standard Edition of the Complete Psychological Works of Sigmund Freud, Volume X (1909): Two Case Histories ("Little Hans" and the "Rat Man")*, 151–318. London: Hogarth.
Freud, S. (1910). A Special Type of Choice of Object Made by Men (Contributions to the Psychology of Love I). In J. Strachey (Ed.), *The Standard Edition of the Complete Psychological Works of Sigmund Freud, Volume XI (1910): Five Lectures on Psycho-Analysis, Leonardo da Vinci and Other Works*, 163–176. London: Hogarth.
Freud, S. (1911a). Formulations on the Two Principles of Mental Functioning. In J. Strachey (Ed.), *The Standard Edition of the Complete Psychological Works of Sigmund Freud, Volume XII (1911–1913): The Case of Schreber Papers on Technique and Other Works*, 213–226. London: Hogarth.
Freud, S. (1911b). Psycho-Analytic Notes on an Autobiographical Account of a Case of Paranoia (Dementia Paranoides). In J. Strachey (Ed.), *The Standard Edition of the Complete Psychological Works of Sigmund Freud, Volume XII (1911–1913): The Case of Schreber Papers on Technique and Other Works*, 1–82. London: Hogarth.

Freud, S. (1913). Totem and Taboo. In J. Strachey (Ed.), *The Standard Edition of the Complete Psychological Works of Sigmund Freud, Volume XIII (1913–1914): Totem and Taboo and Other Works*, vii–162. London: Hogarth.

Freud, S. (1914a). On Narcissism. In J. Strachey (Ed.), *The Standard Edition of the Complete Psychological Works of Sigmund Freud, Volume XIV (1914–1916): On the History of the Psycho-Analytic Movement Papers on Metapsychology and Other Works*, 67–102. London: Hogarth.

Freud, S. (1914b). Some Reflections on Schoolboy Psychology. In J. Strachey (Ed.), *The Standard Edition of the Complete Psychological Works of Sigmund Freud, Volume XIII (1913–1914): Totem and Taboo and Other Works*, 239–244. London: Hogarth.

Freud, S. (1915a). Instincts and Their Vicissitudes. In J. Strachey (Ed.), *The Standard Edition of the Complete Psychological Works of Sigmund Freud, Volume XIV (1914–1916): On the History of the Psycho-Analytic Movement Papers on Metapsychology and Other Works*, 109–140. London: Hogarth.

Freud, S. (1915b). The Unconscious. In J. Strachey (Ed.), *The Standard Edition of the Complete Psychological Works of Sigmund Freud, Volume XIV (1914–1916): On the History of the Psycho-Analytic Movement, Papers on Metapsychology and Other Works*, 159–215. London: Hogarth.

Freud, S. (1916). Some Character-Types Met with in Psycho-Analytic Work. In J. Strachey (Ed.), *The Standard Edition of the Complete Psychological Works of Sigmund Freud, Volume XIV (1914–1916): On the History of the Psycho-Analytic Movement, Papers on Metapsychology and Other Works*, 309–333. London: Hogarth.

Freud, S. (1917a). A Difficulty in the Path of Psycho-Analysis. In J. Strachey (Ed.), *The Standard Edition of the Complete Psychological Works of Sigmund Freud, Volume XVII (1914–1918): From the History of an Infantile Neurosis and Other Works*, 135–144. London: Hogarth.

Freud, S. (1917b). A Metapsychological Supplement to the Theory of Dreams. In J. Strachey (Ed.), *The Standard Edition of the Complete Psychological Works of Sigmund Freud, Volume XIV (1914–1916): On the History of the Psycho-Analytic Movement, Papers on Metapsychology and Other Works*, 217–235. London: Hogarth.

Freud, S. (1917c). Introductory Lectures on Psycho-Analysis. In J. Strachey (Ed.), *The Standard Edition of the Complete Psychological Works of Sigmund Freud, Volume XVI (1916–1917): Introductory Lectures on Psycho-Analysis*, 241–463. London: Hogarth.

Freud, S. (1917d). Mourning and Melancholia. In J. Strachey (Ed.), *The Standard Edition of the Complete Psychological Works of Sigmund Freud, Volume XIV (1914–1916): On the History of the Psycho-Analytic Movement, Papers on Metapsychology and Other Works*, 237–258. London: Hogarth.

Freud, S. (1917e). On Transformations of Instinct as Exemplified in Anal Erotism. In J. Strachey (Ed.), *The Standard Edition of the Complete Psychological Works of Sigmund Freud, Volume XVII (1914–1918): From the History of an Infantile Neurosis and Other Works*, 125–134. London: Hogarth.

Freud, S. (1918). From the History of an Infantile Neurosis. In J. Strachey (Ed.), *The Standard Edition of the Complete Psychological Works of Sigmund Freud, Volume XVII (1917–1919): An Infantile Neurosis and Other Works*, 1–124. London: Hogarth.

Freud, S. (1919a). "A Child Is Being Beaten": A Contribution to the Study of the Origin of Sexual Perversions. In J. Strachey (Ed.), *The Standard Edition of the Complete Psychological Works of Sigmund Freud, Volume XVII (1917–1919): An Infantile Neurosis and Other Works*, 175–204. London: Hogarth.

Freud, S. (1919b). The "Uncanny." In J. Strachey (Ed.), *The Standard Edition of the Complete Psychological Works of Sigmund Freud, Volume XVII (1917–1919): An Infantile Neurosis and Other Works*, 217–256. London: Hogarth.

Freud, S. (1920). Beyond the Pleasure Principle. In J. Strachey (Ed.), *The Standard Edition of the Complete Psychological Works of Sigmund Freud, Volume XVIII (1920): Beyond the Pleasure Principle and Other Works*, 1–64. London: Hogarth.

Freud, S. (1921). Group Psychology and the Analysis of the Ego. In J. Strachey (Ed.), *The Standard Edition of the Complete Psychological Works of Sigmund Freud, Volume XVIII (1920): Beyond the Pleasure Principle and Other Works*, 65–144. London: Hogarth.

Freud, S. (1922). Some Neurotic Mechanisms in Jealousy, Paranoia and Homosexuality. In J. Strachey (Ed.), *The Standard Edition of the Complete Psychological Works of Sigmund Freud, Volume XVIII (1920): Beyond the Pleasure Principle and Other Works*, 221–232. London: Hogarth.

Freud, S. (1923a). A Seventeenth-Century Demonological Neurosis. In J. Strachey (Ed.), *The Standard Edition of the Complete Psychological Works of Sigmund Freud, Volume XIX (1923–1925): The Ego and the Id and Other Works*, 67–106. London: Hogarth.

Freud, S. (1923b). The Ego and the Id. In J. Strachey (Ed.), *The Standard Edition of the Complete Psychological Works of Sigmund Freud, Volume XIX (1923–1925): The Ego and the Id and Other Works*, 1–66. London: Hogarth.

Freud, S. (1924). The Economic Problem of Masochism. In J. Strachey (Ed.), *The Standard Edition of the Complete Psychological Works of Sigmund Freud, Volume XIX (1923–1925): The Ego and the Id and Other Works*, 155–170. London: Hogarth.

Freud, S. (1925). An Autobiographical Study. In J. Strachey (Ed.), *The Standard Edition of the Complete Psychological Works of Sigmund Freud, Volume XX (1925–1926): An Autobiographical Study, Inhibitions, Symptoms and Anxiety, The Question of Lay Analysis and Other Works*, 1–74. London: Hogarth.

Freud, S. (1926a). Inhibitions, Symptoms and Anxiety. In J. Strachey (Ed.), *The Standard Edition of the Complete Psychological Works of Sigmund Freud, Volume XX (1925–1926): An Autobiographical Study, Inhibitions, Symptoms and Anxiety, The Question of Lay Analysis and Other Works*, 75–176. London: Hogarth.

Freud, S. (1926b). The Question of Lay Analysis. In J. Strachey (Ed.), *The Standard Edition of the Complete Psychological Works of Sigmund Freud, Volume XX (1925–1926): An Autobiographical Study, Inhibitions, Symptoms and Anxiety, The Question of Lay Analysis and Other Works*, 177–258. London: Hogarth.

Freud, S. (1927). The Future of an Illusion. In J. Strachey (Ed.), *The Standard Edition of the Complete Psychological Works of Sigmund Freud, Volume XXI (1927–1931): The Future of an Illusion, Civilization and its Discontents, and Other Works*, 1–56. London: Hogarth.

Freud, S. (1930). Civilization and its Discontents. In J. Strachey (Ed.), *The Standard Edition of the Complete Psychological Works of Sigmund Freud, Volume XXI (1927–1931): The Future of an Illusion, Civilization and its Discontents, and Other Works*, 57–146. London: Hogarth.

Freud, S. (1931a). Female Sexuality. In J. Strachey (Ed.), *The Standard Edition of the Complete Psychological Works of Sigmund Freud, Volume XXI (1927–1931): The Future of an Illusion, Civilization and its Discontents, and Other Works*, 221–244. London: Hogarth.

Freud, S. (1931b). Libidinal Types. In J. Strachey (Ed.), *The Standard Edition of the Complete Psychological Works of Sigmund Freud, Volume XXI (1927–1931): The Future of an Illusion, Civilization and its Discontents, and Other Works*, 215–220. London: Hogarth.

Freud, S. (1933). New Introductory Lectures on Psycho-Analysis. In J. Strachey (Ed.), *The Standard Edition of the Complete Psychological Works of Sigmund Freud, Volume XXII (1932–1936): New Introductory Lectures on Psycho-Analysis and Other Works*, 1–182. London: Hogarth.

Freud, S. (1937). Analysis Terminable and Interminable. In J. Strachey (Ed.), *The Standard Edition of the Complete Psychological Works of Sigmund Freud, Volume XXIII (1937–1939): Moses and Monotheism, An Outline of Psycho-Analysis and Other Works*, 209–254. London: Hogarth.

Freud, S. (1938a). An Outline of Psycho-Analysis. In J. Strachey (Ed.), *The Standard Edition of the Complete Psychological Works of Sigmund Freud, Volume XXIII (1937–1939): Moses and Monotheism, An Outline of Psycho-Analysis and Other Works*, 139–208. London: Hogarth.

Freud, S. (1938b). Splitting of the Ego in the Process of Defence. In J. Strachey (Ed.), *The Standard Edition of the Complete Psychological Works of Sigmund Freud, Volume XXIII (1937–1939): Moses and Monotheism, An Outline of Psycho-Analysis and Other Works*, 271–278. London: Hogarth.

Freud, S. (1939). Moses and Monotheism. In J. Strachey (Ed.), *The Standard Edition of the Complete Psychological Works of Sigmund Freud, Volume XXIII (1937–1939): Moses and Monotheism, An Outline of Psycho-Analysis and Other Works*, 1–138. London: Hogarth.

Gilbert, S. & Gubar, S. (1979). *The Madwoman in the Attic: The Woman Writer and the Nineteenth-Century Literary Imagination*. New Haven, CT: Yale University Press.

Green, A. (1997). The Dead Mother. In A. Green, *On Private Madness*, 142–173. London: Karnac (originally published in 1986).

Hendrick, I. (1936). Ego Development and Certain Character Problems. *Psychoanalytic Quarterly*, 5: 320–346.

Herdman, J. (1990). *The Double in Nineteenth-Century Fiction*. New York: Springer.

Hitchcock, A. (Producer & Director). (1960). *Psycho* [Motion Picture]. United States: Paramount Pictures.

Holland, N. (1998) *The Trouble(s) with Lacan*. http://users.clas.ufl.edu/nholland/lacan.htm.

Jackson, P. et al. (Producers) & Jackson, P. (Director). (2003). *The Battle of the Five Armies* [Motion Picture]. New Zealand and United States: Warner Bros. Pictures.

Jackson, P. et al. (Producers) & Jackson, P. (Director). (2012). *An Unexpected Journey* [Motion Picture]. New Zealand and United States: Warner Bros. Pictures.

Jackson, P. et al. (Producers) & Jackson, P. (Director). (2013). *The Desolation of Smaug* [Motion Picture]. New Zealand and United States: Warner Bros. Pictures.

Jackson, R. (1986). Narcissism and Beyond: A Psychoanalytic Reading of *Frankenstein* and Fantasies of the Double. In W. Coyle (Ed.), *Aspects of Fantasy: Selected Essays from the Second International Conference on the Fantastic in Literature and Film*, 45–53. Westport, CT: Greenwood Press.

Jacobson, Edith, 1964: *The Self and Object World*. New York: International Universities Press.

Jameson, F. (2003) Future City. *New Left Review*, 21(May/June): 65–79.

Jones, E. (1926). The Origin and Structure of the Super-Ego. *International Journal of Psychoanalysis*, 7: 303–311.

Jones, E. (1933). The Phallic Phase. *International Journal of Psychoanalysis*, 14: 1–33.

Jones, E. (1953). *The Life and Work of Sigmund Freud*, Vol. 1. New York: Basic Books.

Kardiner, A. (1939). *The Individual and His Society: The Psychodynamics of Primitive Social Organization*. New York: Columbia University Press.

Kavaler-Adler, S. (1993/2013). *The Compulsion to Create: A Psychoanalytic Study of Women Artists*. New York: Routledge.

Kavaler-Adler, S. (1996/2014). *The Creative Mystique: From Red Shoes Frenzy to Love and Creativity*. New York: Routledge.

Kavaler-Adler, S. (2010). Seduction, Date Rape, and Aborted Surrender. *International Forum of Psychoanalysis*, 19(1):15–26.

Kavaler-Adler, S. (2013). Dialectics of Mortality and Immortality: Time as an Internal and Transitional Object Experience and Time as a Persecutory vs. a Holding Object. *MindConsiliums*, 13(12): 1–32.

Keppler, C.F. (1972). *The Literature of the Second Self.* Tucson, AZ: University of Arizona Press.

Klein, M. (1928). Early Stages of the Oedipus Conflict. *International Journal of Psychoanalysis*, 9: 167–180.

Klein, M. (1931). A Contribution to the Theory of Intellectual Inhibition. *International Journal of Psychoanalysis*, 12: 206–218.

Klein, M. (1932). The Psycho-Analysis of Children. *International Psychoanalytic Library*, 22: 1–379. London: Hogarth.

Klein, M. (1935). A Contribution to the Psychogenesis of Manic-Depressive States. *International Journal of Psychoanalysis*, 16: 145–174.

Klein, M. (1940). Mourning and Its Relation to Manic-Depressive States. *International Journal of Psychoanalysis*, 21: 125–153.

Klein, M. (1975). Envy and Gratitude and Other Works 1946–1963. *International Psychoanalytic Library*, 104: 1–346. London: Hogarth and the Institute of Psychoanalysis.

Kohut, H. (1971). *The Analysis of the Self: A Systematic Approach to the Psychoanalytic Treatment of Narcissistic Personality Disorders.* Madison, CT: International Universities Press, 1989.

Kurtz, R. (2007). *Body-Centered Psychotherapy.* Mendocino, CA: LifeRhythm (originally published in 1990).

Lacan, J. (1993). *The Seminar. Book III: The Pscyhoses, 1955–1956.* (R. Grigg, Trans.). London: Routledge.

Lacan, J. (1998). *The Seminar of Jacques Lacan: The Four Fundamental Concepts of Psychoanalysis (Vol. Book XI).* (A. Sheridan, Trans.) New York: Norton.

Lacan, J. (2007). *Écrits: The First Complete Edition in English* (B. Fink, Trans.). New York: Norton (originally published in 1966).

Lampl-De Groot, J. (1947). On the Development of the Ego and Super-Ego. *International Journal of Psychoanalysis*, 28: 7–11.

Lampl-De Groot, J. (1952). Re-Evaluation of the Role of the Oedipus Complex. *International Journal of Psychoanalysis*, 33: 335–342.

Lasker, E. (Producer) & Nyby, C. (Director). (1951). *The Thing from Another World* [Motion Picture]. USA: RKO Radio Pictures.

Lewis, H.B. (1971). *Shame and Guilt in Neurosis.* New York: International Universities Press.

Linson, A., Chaffin, C., Bell, R. (Producers) & Fincher, D. (Director). (1999) *Fight Club* [Motion Picture]. United States and Germany: 20th Century Fox.

Loewald, H.W. (1962). The Superego and the Ego-Ideal. *International Journal of Psychoanalysis*, 43: 264–268.

Lowen, A. (1969). *The Betrayal of the Body.* New York: Macmillan.

Lowen, A. (1994). *Bioenergetics: The Revolutionary Therapy that Uses the Language of the Body to Heal the Problems of the Mind.* New York: Arkana (originally published in 1958).

McDougall, J. (1972). Primal Scene and Sexual Perversion. *International Journal of Psychoanalysis*, 53: 371–384.

McDougall, J. (1974). The Anonymous Spectator: A Clinical Study of Sexual Perversion. *Contemporary Psychoanalysis*, 10: 289–310.

Mackinnon, R.A. & Michels, R. (1971). *The Psychiatric Interview in Clinical Practice.* Philadelphia, PA: W.B. Saunders.

Marx, K. (1844a). *On the Jewish Question.* (Progress Publishers, Trans.). www.marxists.org/archive/marx/works/1844/jewish-question.

Marx, K. (1844b). *The Power of Money* (Progress Publishers, Trans.). www.marxists.org/archive/marx/works/1844/manuscripts/power.htm.

Marx, K. (1845a). *The German Ideology*. (Progress Publishers, Trans.). www.marxists.org/archive/marx/works/1845/german-ideology/ch01a.htm.

Marx, K. (1845b). *Theses on Feuerbach*. (Progress Publishers, Trans.). www.marxists.org/archive/marx/works/1845/theses.

Meissner, W.W. (2008). Self and Time. *Journal of the American Academy of Psychoanalysis and Dynamic Psychiatry*, 36(4): 707–736.

Metz, C. (1982). *The Imaginary Signifier: Psychoanalysis and the Cinema*. Bloomington, IN: Indiana University Press.

Mills, J. (2012). *Conundrums: A Critique of Contemporary Psychoanalysis*. New York: Routledge.

Miyoshi, M. (1969). *The Divided Self: A Perspective on the Literature of the Victorians*. New York: New York University Press.

Mori, M. (2012). The Uncanny Valley (K.F. MacDorman & N. Kageki, Trans.). *IEEE Robotics and Automation*, 19(2): 98–100.

Mulvey, L. (1989). Visual Pleasure and Narrative Cinema. In L. Mulvey, *Visual And Other Pleasures*, 14–26. London: Palgrave Macmillan.

Ogden, P., Minton, K., & Pain, C. (2006). *Trauma and the Body: A Sensorimotor Approach to Psychotherapy* (Norton Series on Interpersonal Neurobiology). New York: W.W. Norton.

Pederson, T. (2015). *The Economics of Libido: Psychic Bisexuality, the Superego, and the Centrality of the Oedipus Complex*. London: Karnac.

Perls, F.S. (1969). *Gestalt Therapy Verbatim*. Moab, UT: Real People Press.

Rank, O. (1941). *Beyond Psychology*. New York: Dover.

Rank, O. (1971). *The Double* (H. Tucker, Jr., Trans.). Chapel Hill, NC: University of North Carolina Press.

Reich, A. (1954). Early Identifications as Archaic Elements in the Superego. *Journal of the American Psychoanalytic Association*, 2: 218–238.

Reich, W. (1990). *Character Analysis*. New York: Farrar, Straus, & Giroux (originally published in 1933).

Richards, A. (2015). Psychoanalysis in Crisis: The Danger of Ideology. *Psychoanalytic Review*, 102(3), 389–405.

Rogers, R. (1970). *A Psychoanalytic Study of the Double in Literature*. Detroit, MI: Wayne State University Press.

Sandler, J. (1960). On the Concept of Superego. *Psychoanalytic Study of the Child*, 15: 128–162.

Shapiro, D. (1999). *Neurotic Styles*. New York: Basic Books.

Shapiro, F. (2001). *Eye Movement Desensitization and Reprocessing: Basic Principles, Protocols, and Procedures*. New York: Guilford Press.

Spotnitz, H. (1969). *Modern Psychoanalysis of the Schizophrenic Patient*. New York: Grune & Stratton.

Stoller, R.J. (1976). Primary Femininity. *Journal of the American Psychoanalytic Association*, 24S (supplement): 59–78.

Tarratt, M. (1986). Monsters from the Id. In Barry Keigh Grant (Ed.), *Film Genre Reader*, 346–365. Austin, TX: University of Texas Press.

Todorov, T. (1973). *Poétique* (Vol. 2). Paris: Éditions du Seuil.

Tran, R. et al. (Producers), Kaufman, C., & Johnson, D. (Directors). (2015). *Anomalisa* [Motion Picture]. United States: Paramount Pictures.

Tustin, F. (1988a). The "Black Hole." *Free Associations*, 1: 35–50.

Tustin, F. (1988b). Psychotherapy with Children who Cannot Play. *International Review of Psychoanalysis*, 15: 93–106.

Tymms, R. (1949). *Doubles in Literary Psychology*. Cambridge, UK: Bowes & Bowes.

Volkan Vamik D. (1997). *Bloodlines: From Ethnic Pride to Ethnic Terrorism*. New York: Farrar, Straus, & Giroux.

Webber, A. (1996). *The Doppelgänger: Double Visions in German Literature*. New York: Oxford University Press.

Winnicott, D.W. (1960). The Theory of the Parent–Infant Relationship. *International Journal of Psychoanalysis*, 41: 585–595.

Žižek, S. (Ed.). (1992). *Everything You Always Wanted to Know About Lacan (But Were Afraid to Ask Hitchcock)*. London: Verso.

INDEX

For Product Safety Concerns and Information please contact our EU representative GPSR@taylorandfrancis.com
Taylor & Francis Verlag GmbH, Kaufingerstraße 24, 80331 München, Germany

www.ingramcontent.com/pod-product-compliance
Ingram Content Group UK Ltd.
Pitfield, Milton Keynes, MK11 3LW, UK
UKHW020141200926
475702UK00005B/849
* 9 7 8 1 1 3 8 3 0 7 0 9 4 *